ON THE BRINGING UP OF
CHILDREN

Founded by C. K. Ogden

The International Library of Psychology

PSYCHOANALYSIS
In 28 Volumes

ON THE BRINGING UP OF CHILDREN

Edited by JOHN RICKMAN

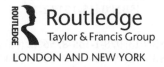

Routledge
Taylor & Francis Group

LONDON AND NEW YORK

First published in 1939
by Routledge
2 Park Square, Milton Park, Abingdon, Oxfordshire OX14 4RN
711 Third Avenue, New York, NY 10017

First issued in paperback 2014

Routledge is an imprint of the Taylor and Francis Group, an informa business

British Library Cataloguing in Publication Data
A CIP catalogue record for this book
is available from the British Library

On the Bringing Up of Children
ISBN 0415-21105-0
Psychoanalysis: 28 Volumes
ISBN 0415-21132-8
The International Library of Psychology: 204 Volumes
ISBN 0415-19132-7

ISBN 13: 978-1-138-87569-2 (pbk)
ISBN 13: 978-0-415-21105-5 (hbk)

CONTENTS

PUBLISHER'S NOTE

SINCE the publication of the First Edition of this book, three of the co-authors, Susan Isaacs, Merell Middlemore, and Ella Sharpe, have died. While the arrangements for the present edition were being completed, the editor, John Rickman, also died suddenly. Mrs Klein therefore undertook to write a brief preface to the Second Edition and to extend the Bibliography to include further important titles. Psycho-analysis has sustained a severe loss by the death of the four members of the profession whose writings have been brought together in this book, but the significance of their work will in no way diminish with the passage of the years, and in fact very little revision has been considered necessary.

PREFACE

THE forces behind the great change in upbringing which took place in the early part of this century were partly scientific, partly social. The researches of Darwin and his contemporaries had produced a new outlook on life; a theory originally concerned with plants and the lower animals penetrated into every branch of biological and social thought, shattered belief in the fixity of species, and in the end revolutionized all ideas of the potentialities of the human species itself. The increased independence of thought among women encouraged them to view their children as persons, who had value and interest because of their potential growth; whereas before there had been a tendency to regard them simply as immature specimens, to be moulded into the likeness of their parents or of the class into which it had pleased God to call them.

When upbringing was in the main traditional rather than scientific, i.e. when it was based on general views as to the proper outlook on the social conventions and not on the observation of individuals, there was no accumulation of knowledge on the subject. In the early years of this century education broke with tradition; teachers became newly observant and helped in the emancipation of childhood by assisting parents to see the way in which the young needed help in this business of growing up, and discipline for discipline's sake was discouraged. But, valuable though this progress was, parents and teachers could not have effected a radical change in outlook in the matter of up-bringing; this followed on the arrival of a new instrument of research which penetrated deeper and farther into the child's mind.

The progress of science and of civilization is frequently held up because the apparatus of research is not flexible enough, or is in other ways inadequate to deal with new problems which arise; scientific concepts may legitimately be included here in the term "apparatus of research," because the dis-tinguishing feature of a scientific concept is that it can be detached from the particular circumstances for which it was first made and be used in other situations that have the same kind of inner relation-ships; and so it comes about that progress in one branch of science enriches and may even revolu-tionize another. Freud's researches were begun on neurotic adults and, in the course of his investiga-tions, he devised a new instrument of research. As always happens under such circumstances, there was immediately a great extension of the field of inquiry, and the outlook on problems apparently unrelated to the original field are revolutionized too.[1] This is what happened in child study.

Observation in the past had been limited to the conscious layers of the mind, the unconscious mental

[1] This happened in the case of Darwin's work, and we may note in passing that not only was it applied in other fields, but that it was misapplied as well.

processes were not discernible; even their existence was in most instances denied. Only recently have we begun to understand the working of the most important components of the child's mind and personality.

The discoveries of psycho-analysis have not of course supplanted the sound work and clear observation already made in education and child welfare, but have given their application greater definition and exactness. They have shown that the growth of the child's mind is a far more complicated process than was once supposed, and that much harm may be done to that growth if a method of upbringing is adopted which underestimates the complexities.

There is nothing to be afraid of in complexity if it is understood; indeed, man has in the long run suffered more from hasty over-simplifications than from confusion over complexities, for over-simplification has led him to assume that he has mastered the problem, when in fact, without knowing it, he has only found refuge in a slogan or a formula.

Tragic instances could be given of parents who have sought advice on problems of upbringing from those who have imperfectly realized the intricacies of the matter they were supposed to be dealing with. Sometimes enthusiasm at the mere fact of a new discovery so takes possession of the mind of the adviser that he omits the rather necessary precaution of thoroughly acquainting himself with the researches in question, and, seeing a part of the new work very vividly, finds satisfaction (and a following) when he preaches and teaches the new doctrine, not realizing that, unless he has grasped the problem as a whole, he runs grave danger of misleading those who put their trust in him. Psycho-analysis has suffered much from enthusiastic followers who do not follow close enough, and to demand that those who pretend to use it should know what they are talking about is not unreasonable. It is neither possible nor desirable for practitioners to follow up each misrepresentation of facts or distortion of a valuable scientific theory with a denial or an explanation. Science unfortunately cannot prevent misapplication of its discoveries or distortion of its theories, but the spread of knowledge should in the end reduce the damage done by misguided enthusiasts.

One of the conclusions drawn by those who have not grasped the real implications of " the new psychology " is that if a child were properly brought up he would have no nervous difficulties, and that the prevalence of nervous troubles is proof that parents are always doing the wrong thing to their offspring. This is not only untrue but it has made upbringing much more difficult for the conscientious parent.

To put all the blame on parents for the neurotic ills of their children is not only unfair to parents, but is a disservice to the children, because it tends to obscure the importance of the child's own intricate mental activities and to regard him as a piece of inactive plastic material. There are inherent difficulties in mental adjustment which are liable to cause trouble however good the home; the child's sense of guilt is one of these, and if that is ignored we are not in a position to help him to lessen that guilt. Besides, if the parents always assume that something they have done has made the child nervous, they tend to look for some recent and specific act of their own as its cause, and they become nervous themselves and fear to exert any parental influence at all in the development of their children.

The really important factor in upbringing is the *general attitude* of the parents, and the way in which the *ordinary details* of life are conducted. The crises and decisions, which occupy so much time in parents' meetings and informal discussions, are of much less significance. For example, a decision to inflict no corporal punishment may in itself be admirable, but unless this is supported by an understanding of the child's attitude towards its own misdemeanours the good intention which gave rise to the decision will be of no avail, for in avoiding corporal punishment the parents may overlook the harmful effects of a moralizing attitude, so that the child will grow up with an exaggerated sense of guilt and moral responsibility.

Things which seem trivial to the parents may be of vast importance to the child. The little liberties and restrictions are often details about which his fantasy life is much occupied, though to the grown-up who does not understand his fantasies they seem small. On the other hand, points which seem important to the parents, clean hands and good table manners, for instance, should be allowed to grow in significance for the child rather than be thrust upon him as a duty. It is as unreasonable to expect of children a uniformity of social growth as to expect them to add the same number of inches each year to their height. The acquisition of good manners is not always rapid, and they are not always well founded if too quickly acquired. The capacity to make good contact with other people and retain an easy relation with them is more important than the capacity to imitate their behaviour; in no case is this good contact of more importance than in the relation between parent and child; it enables the child to build up a strong and flexible personality, independent and self-reliant but retaining an affection for the older generation which will add depth and warmth to the welcome which awaits a yet younger one.

There is one topic to be referred to later on in this book which commonly receives less attention than its due—namely, the rôle of the father in upbringing. The position of the mother is never lost sight of, the father's is more obscure but almost as important. In his fantasies the child gives about an equal attention to father and mother figures, so fathers have no real ground for feeling out of the picture, as many do. It is true that children are often more demonstrative to their mothers, but our knowledge of the child's fantasies now enables us to penetrate beneath the surface and to see that great interest is directed to the father even if it is not shown. Once during a public discussion on upbringing I heard a man ask rather wistfully whether the father had any other function than that of a friendly background in the home. In the past the question would not have been easy to answer, but we know enough to-day to frame the outline of a reply.

The child always pictures himself as *vis-à-vis* both his father and mother; the triangular relationship may or may not be harmonious in these fantasies, but it is never—even in orphans—a concept of mother and son, mother and daughter, without some trace of a father figure. Children need to see the interplay of personality of father and mother, male and female, for their social imagination is far more active than is generally realized, and they are helped by observing the friendliness of one sex to the other. If the father and mother are at loggerheads it will be hard for the child to envisage with satisfaction the founding of a home of his own, whereas the experience of a congenial home fosters the desire to produce a similar one for oneself. He needs to see the considerate behaviour of his parents to óne another, their good humour in the face of vexation, their camaraderie, and a mutual loyalty, for by these observations the child is strengthened in a belief that he can overcome his own jealousies and aggression, his inconsiderateness, ill humour and perfidiousness.

But the father has a more particular and personal rôle to perform. The child's sensitiveness feels the difference between the man's outlook on life and the woman's, appreciates that the father understands his needs and can give him help in a different way from the mother. (The child quickly sees that in the matter of affection, courage, delicacy and moral strength there is nothing to choose between the male and the female in spite of the enormous differences in other ways, and that their approaches to life are complementary. Consolation in grief or suffering, punishment, or virtues such as endurance should not be associated in the mind of the child with either sex alone.)

In the child's mind there is, besides the picture of a strict and punishing father, the conception of the father who is the embodiment of creativeness, and is the skilled adviser who helps little children out of their difficulties. If the father really gives help, this encourages the child's confidence in others and increases his capacity to co-operate with people outside the home when he grows up (this applies also to the mother, of course).

All kinds of fantasies are present in the child's mind, the atmosphere of the home influences the development of those which determine whether the disposition towards the world shall be a friendly one or a hostile one. So the answer to the plaintive query from the man at the public lecture takes two directions : the first is that the father is in the foreground *vis-à-vis* the mother, and so gives a prevision of the child's own married life ; the second, not unconnected with the first, is that the father is seen in the rôle of a stimulating producer of good things, chief among these being other children ; whether the child is a boy or a girl this concept will be equally important, though of course from different aspects.

I should perhaps say something about the genesis of this book. To meet an increasingly pressing demand for some statement on upbringing from the psycho-analytical standpoint, a public lecture course was arranged in the Spring of 1935.[1] It was not a systematic course but a selection of topics which were of special interest to the lecturers. The demand for the lectures in book form led to their revision for publication. The editor has eliminated repetition as far as seemed to him expedient, but when points are brought up in different contexts in such a way as to throw further light on the problems, they are better all left in.

In conclusion I want to say a word about what has been called the intrusion of science into the home. Some people contend that parental instinct is a sufficient guide to upbringing, an expression of the general notion that there is something incompatible between the exercise of intuition and the possession of conscious knowledge. I believe this to be a serious error. Since science is intellectual, it cannot claim the last word in the guidance of human affairs, but just because it is based on reason, it must have the next to last word. No amount of thinking can take the place of love, and if the emotional attitude is not right, it is hard for the intellectual side to keep a good balanced outlook on the world.

Wherein does the change lie between the upbringing of the past and the present? Goodwill there has always been, but there was ignorance about the very important deep levels of the child's mind.

[1] The general title was " Can Upbringing be Planned ? " The order of the lectures has been changed, but otherwise the arrangement and content is substantially the same.

The instrument of investigation first devised by Freud for dealing with adults, and developed later by Mrs. Klein for application to children, has radically changed our outlook, and has made it safer to embark on the responsibility of upbringing, by making us less dependent on the sometimes wise but always rather blind guidance of tradition.   The new researches have done more for us than add to our intellectual knowledge, they have given us an insight into the mind of the young child which has deepened our emotional and living understanding of that all-important bond—the relation between parent and child.

J. R.

11 Kent Terrace,
  Regent's Park,
   London, N.W.1.
    January 26th, 1936.

PREFACE
TO THE SECOND EDITION

THE essays contained in this volume are based on psycho-analytic experience and theory. It therefore seems appropriate to consider the progress of psycho-analytic knowledge in the years which have elapsed since 1936. There has been a more general acceptance of certain findings which are embodied in this book, above all of the fundamental importance of aggressive impulses and fantasies and their part in the causation of anxiety and guilt. This implies also a growing recognition that depressive feelings and the tendency to make reparation originate in early infancy. There is a second trend of development which occurs to me as particularly noteworthy, namely, further research into the earliest stage of the infant's development.

Except for a few additions to the bibliography and a short postscript, this book is being reprinted without alteration. In my view, the passage of years has not in any way deprived it of its original merit.

MELANIE KLEIN

LONDON.
January, 1952.

xvii

I. PLANNING FOR STABILITY

BY ELLA FREEMAN SHARPE

PSYCHO-ANALYSIS has hitherto only offered negative
advice in the matter of the upbringing of children,
what *not* to do rather than what to do. Can psycho-
analytical research offer a positive contribution,
suggest a plan for upbringing that will ensure
mental health? In subsequent chapters, others
from their intimate experiences will discuss with
regard to specific problems whether or not, or to
what extent, it is possible to proceed on a pre-
conceived plan. This leaves me free to deal with
basic principles that psycho-analytical research
reveals. However the accent of our research may
shift as hitherto unknown factors emerge or old
ones take on new significance, fundamentals remain
unshakable.

The greatest contribution psycho-analysis has
made to social science is that it reveals the possibility of greater self-knowledge, knowledge of
the hidden self and the dynamics of the unconscious
mind. The implications of that fact are so vast,
that Freud may one day be looked upon as the first
real guardian of a natural morality, a morality
infinitely more profound and integrated than any
so far evolved. For only out of more deep-going

self-knowledge can emerge more rational self-control and fuller personal development. The social reformer's task lies in the external scene of social misery and menace of war. 'The psycho-analyst's task lies primarily with the individual, " Man, know thyself ". Yet external social problems are inseparable from the internal and individual ones. The problem of war will not be solved until individuals have recognized and utilized their own aggressive impulses. Only through the courageous mental and emotional struggles of individuals towards the attainment of self-knowledge and objectivity can there be evolved a body of positive teaching on the subject of training of children and a knowledge of what constitutes the most propitious environment for children's upbringing.

It is easy enough to recognize that we are born into an organized social' community, and that unless we are to be outlawed or imprisoned we must fit into or adapt ourselves to it, in the course of growing up. So with the individual's first community, the home, there is a pattern in being into which the baby is born, and to which he must orientate himself. This community embraces the personalities of the parents, their relationship to each other and the atmosphere of the home created by them. There is a fundamental pattern of behaviour in this individual community which constitutes a most vital factor in the baby's upbringing. In the first months the baby's life is lived in closest union with the mother. The mother's spontaneous emotional relationship

to her child is of incalculable moment, and all
conscious planning falls into second place of importance.

I said " personality " rather than character.
There is a difference. A person may be in adult
respects an admirable character if we are considering
virtues that are socially valuable such as honesty
and strength of will. Such character traits are
nevertheless compatible with lack of imagination
and hardness of heart. It is personality that counts
for the baby, the whole person emotionally, not the
crystallized virtues of adult character. This implicit
pattern of behaviour in a woman is not called out
to its depth until she has a child, but it is possible
for those who can read the signs to foreshadow
what this will be. There is evoked from the
mother an emotional pattern which forms the
setting to which the baby will make its first psychical
reactions, and whether we like it or not, it is not
what we say, nor what we *plan*, but what we *are* in
total personality that matters. There are parents
who through ignorance make many mistakes in
the details of handling children, and yet the children
ride triumphantly over them. There are parents
who through conscious knowledge can avoid
making these same mistakes, but whose children
nevertheless turn out failures.

The implicit pattern evoked in the mother is at
the moment my consideration. I will give you
examples from my own analytical researches. I
have found that a mother's attitude to her child is
profoundly influenced by her unconscious reactions
to her mother, or father. The situation is, so to

speak, reversed. If there exists in her, still un-resolved, her own childhood's angers and resent-ments against her own mother, her attitude to her baby is not and cannot be what we fain would like to imagine, a new pure joy at creation. The mother's emotions contain all her own past; that past can exert its influence in such ways as these: the woman who has made strong reaction-forma-tions, or repressed the unconscious hostility to her mother, will treat manifestations of anger and rage in children with non-understanding severity; more than that, a child's peccadilloes will be regarded as enormities. In other words, she is afraid of the manifestation of infantile anger, since she is still afraid in her unconscious mind of those same infantile manifestations of anger against her own mother. The pattern repeats itself. For example, the mother who reacts to a child who has spilled water with a vehemence only justified if the child were going to drown her, is acting in terms not only of the child's unconscious *momentary* wish, but in terms also of her own anxiety concerning that very same wish in her own unconscious mind. She is afraid not only of the child's aggression but her own, and the child knows it, and this again increases the child's own fear of its power.

Take another type of manifestation of unresolved hostility. A strong reaction to infantile aggression often finds expression in over-solicitude concerning health. This is the unconscious difficulty that besets a mother who is over-anxious concerning the health of the baby. Every sign that all is not well

4

is magnified into a threat of death. To put it plainly, she has to be ever on her guard lest her unconscious hostility should bring disaster to the child she loves. As a result she develops an anxious fussiness that never allows the child to be at peace, and the child will react to this in many untoward ways. The child knows unconsciously what this constant interference means, even though its knowledge is inarticulate.

Dislike of feeding the baby at the breast, or a functional inability to do so is, I have found, ultimately always determined by profound psychological reactions on the mother's part, mainly to unconscious fear of the baby being a hostile or aggressive object, this fear arising from the mother's own unresolved aggression. I have known children to be sent from home to boarding-school at the earliest possible moment. No matter what the ostensible reasons were, analysis of the mother of such children revealed the mother's fear of her own unconscious hostility and consequently a need to save both herself and her children from mutual unconscious aggression. Mothers who thrust their babies as soon as possible upon nurses and servants are under the dominance of these same unconscious anxieties. Economic reasons may be put forward against this, but these do not concern me in this chapter. We are dealing here with mental forces which all too readily fall in with and exploit the custom of foster-nursing. When women want to nurse and bring up their own children they will do so and make the conditions fit their wishes. The women who hand over their children more or less entirely to other people [1] do so for the same reason as those who send them away prematurely to school—namely, those unresolved emotions which arose first of all in relation to their own parents, who may of course have been every whit as much involved themselves. The blame lies nowhere and the need for understanding everywhere. Psycho-analysis says in effect that if a start is to be made at all it must begin with oneself.

Let us now turn to the actual environmental setting in which the parents are the most important figures. From my own analytical practice, mainly among adults, I can say that when a baby passes through infancy to childhood in an environment where the parents have a stabilized happy relationship there is an explicit pattern which will be interwoven in the child's psychic life, and whatever the child's psychic problems may be, this at least will be a factor ever making for normality.

There comes a time in every child's development when his future is determined by the nature and power of his identification. Given an infancy not

---

[1] The nurse of course may actually be a superior person to the mother in the matter of emotional adjustments. The mother then need not be surprised if her son marries a woman of so-called lower class, any more than a woman who sends her child away too early to school need be surprised if her child as it grows up prefers any other place to home. On the other hand, the most efficient nurse may pursue methods with the child that the mother's conscious attitude would deplore. The implicit plan that exposes children to a haphazard emotional environment is the outcome of unresolved emotional problems in the parents.

too anxiety-ridden, the boy passes on to desire to be like his father and the girl to be like her mother, and the fulfilment of those wishes in adult life will be helped or hindered according to whether or no it seems to be a happy thing to be married and have a husband and children as mother has, or to be married and have a wife and home as father has. Hence the explicit environmental plan is of great importance. If the biological urges are attended by knowledge of parental unhappiness in their actual fulfilment, there is, added to all the unconscious factors that make for conflict in children, another one which may make the individual problems of a child well-nigh unsolvable.

If there are children already in the milieu into which the child is born, the organized routine on which the children's lives is run is one into which the child must fit himself and react in terms of himself as an individual. A child quickly learns, when authority is divided, that appeal can be made from one parent to another. If one parent is obdurate, he can, when there is no unity in the home, bend the other to his will. He quickly finds out the difference in treatment given to a favoured child when there is conscious or unconscious preference.

In some homes the eldest remains a privileged person all the time. On the other hand, there are homes where every privilege is given to baby, who is kept helpless as long as possible, so that jealousy is fostered and the pleasure in getting older is spoiled by the fact that the parents evidently preferred immaturity. We need not be surprised if

7

things go wrong when these same children grow up and are expected to take over the responsibilities of adult life.

Explicit plans that are consciously adopted without any reference to the individual child should come under scrutiny—for example, assuming responsibility for· determining the child's future career. This occurs most frequently when traditional family careers weigh heavily, so that as a matter of course the army, the navy, the bar, are allotted to the children, often in that very order, and the child is shaped to fit the necessary education. I have known boys sent to the navy as cadets, who not only have hated their whole training, but who have been sea-sick off and on all through those years. It was one long period of apprehension and misery and yet they were too terrified of their parents to protest.

There are explicit plans adopted other than those dictated by the parents' ambition or family tradition. From time to time new revolutionary educational schemes are promulgated. The absolutely " free " school where children " do just what they want " without let or hindrance was one such revolution. Parents in the flood of revolt against the stultifying effects of hard discipline and repression hailed such " free " schools as the salvation of children and the ushering in of a new era. But though the old was wrong the reaction was not therefore right. It was the swing of a pendulum.

Scientific feeding and upbringing of the child, the regulation of times, length and number of feeds can be adopted. But all these plans can go astray when applied irrespective of the individual child and when they have not been submitted to the intelligent and above all the loving scrutiny of the parents. The awareness on the parents' part of the possibility of unconscious hostility to the children they love should make them look into their own motives before subjecting children to plans and experiments. Even the plan of scientific feeding, based on most creditable physiological experience, when adhered to in a hard and obdurate manner can itself be pernicious if the individual child and its anxieties are not taken into account.

So far I have dealt with my theme by indicating that there are plans already in being into which the child must fit. There is the most fundamental pattern of behaviour made by the personalities of the parents, whose wise or unwise, positive or ambivalent attitude to the children will be of first importance. There is the actual environmental plan, the happy or unhappy relationship of the parents, and divided or united authority. There is the nursery community and the problem of preference for youngest or oldest, for boy or girl. There are the consciously made decisions for the future of the child, the more pernicious where children are drilled into obedience, and fear of the parents rules. Finally I have indicated the bias of the parents in adopting, either through enthusiasm or conscious reason, plans for upbringing or education without any examination of such plans in the light of the individuality of the child, or investigation into their own motives for adopting such measures.

9

In the same way personal unconscious factors may be just as responsible for the parents refusing to call in assistance from others lest it interfere with the plans which have been " decided on as best " for the child. There exist experts, medical, psychological and educational, whose experience every parent upon occasion needs. The adoption of suggestions made by these experts will often lead to a better relationship between parents and children. Parents who are able to scrutinize their own unconscious minds will avoid two extreme courses—namely, either of shifting the total responsibility of their children's welfare upon the expert or of refusing to consider the advice the experts can give.

I propose next to indicate the lines upon which conscious plans for upbringing can be based in the light of psycho-analytical research. Details will be found in later chapters, but I would say now that only those plans that take cognizance of certain facts will bring good results as wished. The first fact is that if the baby survives at all he will have to go through many stages of development, physical and psychical, which we all have had to go through in our progress from complete dependence to maturity of independence. We must picture what that development would be under ideal conditions. This is important because only so can parents themselves preserve an elasticity of adjustment to the different needs of the child at different times. We can put the matter in this way : do the parents want the child to develop its own potentialities, or do they simply want him to become an extension or fulfilment of their own

ambitions and dreams? I believe that individuality starts very early and the sooner Ann becomes
Ann, and not " baby ", the more propitious is her
future. The Ann-ness of Ann is something the
parents will have to recognize sooner or later, and
the sooner this is done the easier it will be for Ann
and her parents also.

The child is subjected to two factors which will
greatly affect his development: the first is his
physical environment, the second is the psychical.
Taking the physical conditions first, we have in the
last two generations begun to recognize the value
of health, and the interrelation of this to mental
satisfaction in life, but we have yet some way to go
before we realize fully the part played by the
sensuous pleasures and responses in a healthy
attitude to the world around us. Dr. Middlemore
will deal with this at greater length. I want here
to put forward only one point—that the psychical
contact with the environment (what we mean by
a " grasp " on things) is a process which has
momentum. A child whose sensuous life suffers
severe checks at the start, whose emotional life
is subject to unnecessary conflicts, is handicapped
in getting under weigh, and reaches adolescence
(the period when sources of pleasure and of conflict
are more localized) with less power of enjoyment
and less capacity to give it. Children must be
allowed to develop their own momentum of
sensuous pleasure in themselves and their own
environment and to find their own goals.

We are more likely to be successful with psychical
problems if we fully realize the importance of this

intricate physical one, especially if we recognize it early in life, for we find that psychical life is healthy only as it approximates to this ideal of development. I can best illustrate by a remark of a patient of mine a few days ago. She had been in some anxiety thinking how she could bring about certain changes that were evidently necessary in her work. " Chaos," she said, " the thing is in chaos." Then she breathed a sigh of relief and said, " Well, there's plenty of time in which to do my work. There's really no hurry. Better let a plan evolve itself slowly like that hyacinth, than adopt one in a hurry." She pointed to a hyacinth that for days had been slowly unfolding its buds. Not only was her remark profoundly true with regard to all true creative work, but its profundity is based upon physical laws which have their counterpart in the psychical. What I want particularly to stress is the disturbances in the *rate* of psychical growth, as well as of the growth itself, which occurs when the ambitions and anxieties of parents impinge on the child's own as yet unstable equilibrium, and throw it out of its natural rate and mode of growth and its natural internal co-ordination.

Our first aim should be to recognize the physical pattern already in being, and our orientation must be to the individual child. We must not thwart nature. Our personal prejudices derived from the unconscious, our anxieties and our ignorances spoil nature's plan and complicate the problems due to the mixture of love and hate impulses with which the child has to deal early in life. These are more difficult to manage in infancy because impulses are then operating in an immature and over-plastic organism.

Mrs. Klein will tell about the extraordinary adjustments which a baby has to make, physically and psychically, in the first year or so of its life; what I want to emphasize now is that we must recognize the kind of interference which is likely to interrupt orderly development. I will enumerate a few. Excessive stimuli of light and noise; the distraction of new people and their attentions; exaggerated parental efforts to evoke responses of affection or intelligence; the urging of effort of any kind before the child can easily accomplish it; too frequent changes of environment before the child has mastered previous ones; too strict adherence to set rules concerning feeding and keeping the child clean, as for example the insistence on waking of children out of deep sleep to make them pass water. Also a succession of different nurses between infancy and the age of four or five, if such nurses have the entire charge of a child, has the most serious effect upon such a child's development. First of all this means an unstable environment when the child itself is at its most unstable period physically and emotionally and needs the support of environmental steadiness. Secondly, in addition to the temperamental changes that a succession of nurses introduce into the nursery, the varying standards of behaviour this often entails, the changes of habit routine are bewildering and disintegrating to a child who is already in the throes of problems of adjustment.

These are some of the interferences with orderly

development which are preventable, but, the most pernicious of all, is the endeavour to *force* the rate of growth, and of adaptation to grown-up standards. To urge children to turn into little men and women is a violation of a natural process conditioned by the child's own inherent powers and difficulties. By rate of growth I mean a sequence of unfoldment, of development such as the patient to whom I referred earlier realized as she watched daily the slow flowering of the hyacinth.

There is one other situation of major importance in this connection, namely, that of allowing the infant to sleep in the same room as the parents. In every case but one in my experience it was clear that the child had at some time or other been present during parental intercourse, and many problems of anxiety centre around this experience. Now on dispassionate analysis of these anxieties one could not say that a baby who has never been in the parents' bedroom will thereby be saved from the conflicts which are aroused by such early experiences, for these conflicts arise in every case because they are expressions of an innate instability; but analysis shows that the way in which the child achieves stability is in part determined by the way in which his emotional instability has been handled on these occasions. If the baby is awakened out of sleep by sounds made by the parents, he will, in the anxiety of the moment and in the crying which expresses the anxiety, need to be pacified by the mother's turning her attention to him. A first disturbance of this kind, if followed by frequent repetitions, sets up a pattern of behaviour which parents should remember may have an untoward influence on the child's subsequent emotional development.

A quick relief of the infant's anxiety by attending to it will naturally mitigate matters on a first occasion, but every subsequent repetition of the maternal attention lays down more firmly a habit for the infant. The need for reassurance in the face of inner disturbance (which produces the anxiety) leads the child to demand its mother, and this disturbing of the parents leads to a new source of apprehension. This is one reason why children develop night terrors and so often insist on returning to the parents' room. Again, I am not saying that this is the only reason, nor that a child who has never been disturbed will not have night terrors, but I am saying that a child who has been disturbed in its sleep and awakened by the parents time after time will have experienced more exacerbation of anxiety and will have had its aggressive impulses aroused to a greater degree than it can deal with, and far more than it should be called upon to manage. Moreover, I have found in my analytical work that where a child suffered during long periods from night terrors and later in life from insomnia, he or she in infancy had always undergone this cycle of experience.

I am not condemning parents for letting children sleep in their room, still less am I condemning the children for waking up fretful or angry. I want to point out that when parents arrange their household (for financial or other reasons) so that their children share their room, they must realize that they may be angrily disturbed, and that the child's anger and disturbance needs the most careful handling. They should ask themselves whether such bedroom sharing is unavoidable. Sleep is vital to a baby, disturbance is always bad; such jealousy-provoking disturbances are doubly so.

Any interference with bodily functioning that is too frequent or prolonged will set up psychophysical problems in later years; even the well-meant, repeated administration of enemata, ear syringing for wax, nasal douching, and other medical remedies should be brought into question, and the parent should ask the family medical adviser as to when such remedial interferences may be given up, as well as when they should be started. The too-long continuance of these practices are due to over-anxiety in the parents, who should ask themselves whether there are not other ways of dealing with the trouble that confronts them. Apart from the psychical disturbances, the interference with bodily function may itself be serious. The chain of reflexes concerned in defæcation should be disturbed as little as possible by mechanical or chemical means.

I have referred to interference with the gradual unfolding and development of the child, which acts by retarding or accelerating its rate of growth. I will now turn to those disturbances of psychical growth which are due to a parental plan or outlook that disregards or thwarts the child's natural development.

I can illustrate best by an actual example. A

patient said, " My mother only cared that I should be neat and tidy and behave myself nicely when I came down for tea in the drawing-room. She never cared about what went on in my mind." Here you see that the impression left on the child of its upbringing is all on one note, that of being clean, tidy and well-behaved. Unfortunately that impression was correct. Add to this that the entire washing and cleaning of the baby was done by a nurse, and that she was never handled by the mother except when clean, and you will understand how it is that this young woman has very mixed feelings towards children and that her main occupation is keeping her house neat and tidy. That is to say, the mother's own attitude was a positive hindrance to the development of psychical interests other than those associated with neatness, tidiness and good behaviour. The fact is that disturbances in the capacity to make adaptation and to enjoy life always occur when parents have regarded their children as simply objects to be trained and kept in order and, later, to be educated. Only where they have been appreciated as psychical entities with an intense emotional life of their own can adaptation be made. The assumption that children are too small, too young, and above all too ignorant never helps at all. They chafe at being small, they resent being too young, above all they hate being ignorant. Half the environmental difficulties in education arise from the superior attitude of the grown-up who gives to the child the impression that he is ignorant and so must be taught (and at the same time is constantly intimating that there are things that he ought not to know).[1] We do not attempt to teach the child his own language. We do not say, " Here is something of which you are ignorant and you must learn." The child " picks up " language by listening, and when he utters his first intelligible word the listeners applaud. Parents do not feel any anxiety about his learning to speak except where there is an organic reason; when they take it for granted the child finds himself talking in due course. When parents are over-solicitous, or when they take up a mocking tone at the child's blunders as some parents actually do, then the child finds it hard to establish an identification with the fluently speaking, long-admired grown-up, and his acquisition of speech is hindered. Even worse, his confidence in his capacity to grow up is impaired.

We should do well to remember this in connection with other things than language. The acquisition of attainments such as good manners and desirable habits comes through imitation and identification (the former is a more conscious, the latter an unconscious process), and we find that children who have been brought up in an environment where the parents were courteous to each other and treated their children with equal courtesy have less difficulty in making effective emotional contact with their environment.

We can help or hinder the child in the tasks he

[1] The task the teacher is faced with when a child is nervously inhibited is that of obtaining the child's own sanction to the acquisition of knowledge, and so of mobilizing its own energies and developing its innate abilities.

has inevitably to face in his development, we cannot do them for him, either on the psychical or physical plane : but if we understand his problem we can make it easier for him to obtain a better grasp of his difficulties and help to a better outcome. The first point we have to bear in mind is the primitive nature of the baby's mind, its lack of knowledge of how things actually exist and are carried on, of how and why anything is done to it. At first it does not even realize that its body is its own. Its life begins at its mouth, and all its development, bodily and psychical, will radiate and amplify from that mouth experience. The mouth and nipple situation unites the two great instincts of self-preservation and love, which are the dynamics that will supply the energy for every activity, physical and psychical, until life ends. The baby, with its complete ignorance of reality, has one basic experience from which will grow its ability to deal efficiently with the external world, namely, happy, care-free sucking. This is the first act of co-ordination, the first sensuous contact with another person, the first act of union; when this relationship is consolidated in the baby's experience it is ready for progress to other and more creative achievements.

The acquisition of stability and confidence comes slowly, but when we consider the raw material of instincts which the child has first to deal with in his formative years, the cultural achievement of even a three-year-old is astonishing. At first the baby can experience only states of pleasure and pain. Painful stimuli from without, increase of tension within, are regarded as threats to its being which are inflicted on it by the environment and are reacted to accordingly. One must remember its lack of time sense, its lack of experience. It has no knowledge that the tension will eventually be relieved, that the pain will pass, nor does it realize at first that if the breast is not given when it wants it that it will ever come back at all. The endurance of delay is learned slowly, because painful anxiety hinders a comprehension of the orderliness of the world.

Psycho-analysis has discovered that anxiety, associated with aggression, is, even in very young children, accompanied by fantasies which express the turbulent emotions and confused and unstable contact with the environment characteristic of their stage of development. Some people are horrified to hear that children have terrifying fantasies : they half realize this truth and it frightens them. We grown-ups have a more or less strongly stabilized reality sense, we distinguish the real from the imagined, in fantastic things like a Mickey Mouse film in which there is wholesale explosion and chaos, or when we see Charlie Chaplin, in delirium caused by hunger, imagining his friend turning into a hen which he is about to kill. We know that even in the Klondyke Gold Rush friends are not killed and eaten. A child " imagines " that such things happen and the dreadful possibility (for such it becomes in the child's mind since he has not this reality sense) arouses horror. It comes to dread some of its own impulses, and seeks help from without to check its violence. Aggressive thoughts are thus one of the causes of a dependent attitude in the child. One of the strings it ties about itself is love, the other is the fear of its own aggression. The parent who ties the child in leading strings is himself dominated unconsciously by the same fantasies that terrify the child.

To know such facts and to understand the processes of the child's mind seems to me most desirable, it reduces the harmfulness of a rigid parental plan for the child and in addition makes the task of upbringing easier: anxiety holds up parent and child alike. But we must not forget that there are anxieties and conflicts which can never be spared the child. Sooner or later parent and child have to realize that nipple and comforter should be given up and that His Majesty the baby must abdicate his throne, he may have to give up being the only child, he will have to give up "first place" with his mother. By our imaginative understanding of his nature and the adaptation of our plans to his need we can foster growth and reduce the period of "childish" behaviour. The situations I have just mentioned are the most poignant crises in life; emotional crises in adult life arrange themselves on old patterns and we tend to deal with them successfully or unsuccessfully according as we reacted to similar situations in our own childhood.

The close connection between physical and psychical should guide us in the matter of measuring psychical adjustment, for just as the body cannot be made to grow at more than a few inches a year, so mental development has its own rate.

Those who plan for rapid progress run the risk of stunting or retarding growth. But although I have been speaking of physical and psychical growth as if they were merely good analogies, I must remind you that the measure of psychical growth is not just the yard-stick of adult " good behaviour ". The development I speak of is an increase of stability in an unstable system. We must be prepared to meet disturbances of the child's equilibrium without losing our own.

Some changes in environment call for great readjustment of emotions : for example, the birth or death of a brother or sister. The work of adjustment will be greater if the stimuli are large, or if several come at the same time, or in such quick succession that there is no opportunity to regain stability from one before the next disturbance arrives. A child who has to undergo an operation at the same time as the mother is expecting another baby is meeting two massive stimuli at the same time, either of which alone might be borne without shock. A child who loses a sister or brother or parent has to make a massive psychical adjustment. We are accustomed to think that the younger the child the less it is affected by these events ; but that leaves out of account the influence of the fantasy life. The younger the child the more it will be a prey to its own fantastic dreads and fears. In the analysis of an adult, I found that the problems of his later years crystallized in a trauma received when he was four. On one and the same walk with his Nannie he saw a man fall dead at his feet from a high ladder and, before he reached home, he saw his own little dog run over. If a child has measles we call in a doctor. The time will come, one hopes, when we shall have imagination enough to call in a psychologist when a child has to make extensive psychological adjustments to events of this nature.

A boy's father died when the boy is three. Friends of the family and his relations talked to him even at that early age of his taking his father's place, of looking after his mother and being her consolation. Thirty years later analysis proved that at that age he thought he *ought* to take his father's place, a task psychically as well as physically beyond his powers. As a man he was still dealing with this demand fixed at the age of three. Parents who thrust their emotional unhappiness too much on their children are giving them burdens they are not equal to bearing; this applies especially in those cases where a child's aggressiveness has been unusually strong. The child is sensitive to the unhappiness of the parents and feels the burden doubly great when it is coping with feelings of guilt born of its own aggression, for it believes that the domestic unhappiness is due to its own bad thoughts and impulses. A mother's or father's unhappiness will add to every one of the child's psychical problems.

Knowledge of sexual development is needed if wise planning is to be possible. The Freudian discovery of infantile sexuality horrified the conventional moralist, yet no thinking person knowing anything of adult life could fail to recognize that what is oftenest wrong with sexuality in adults is

its infantility.   It is in fact these immature forms of
sexuality which excite the most horror and their
existence is often denied where immaturity is
normal, namely, in children.

Sexual development begins in infancy, not at
adolescence.   The discovery of this was hindered
by fear in the past, and fear makes many blind
to-day, but Freud's original discovery concerning
infantile sexuality has been proved beyond all question.   Genital sensations, erection in the male and
vaginal excitement in the female, occur in infancy.
Only by the retention of and development of the
early sexual orientation in male and female will
biological and psychical maturity be attained : vicis-
situdes in development that lead to diminution or
too great repression of the sexual instinct, or change
in its aim, will cripple and deform it in later life.
A happy sexual union with cheerful acceptance of
its responsibility, with the necessary giving and
serving on the part of both partners, is an all too rare
achievement.   A full accommodation to the sexual
situation, psychical and physical, is too often an
ideal towards which men and women struggle but
do not attain.   Our need is not less sexuality, but
a flowering of it.

Civilization, by demanding a long period of non-
fulfilment, places a burden on our adolescents, who
have to defer, perhaps for years, the gratification of
sexual aims for which they are sexually mature
enough at, say, fifteen or sixteen.   It may be that
some of the discontent with our civilization is
due to the fact that though society winks at incon-
tinence it does nothing to assist youth to bear the

burden of frustration; perhaps one of the reasons why the new civilization in Russia, which in many ways seems to us strange and harsh, is acceptable to the youth of that country is because obstacles are not put by the social and economic system in the way of those who wish to start early on married and family life.

It is the psychical manifestation of sexual energy in sublimation to which we owe civilization, and the important thing to realize is that it is not repression of this energy, but utilization of it, which will make a child interested in the external world. It is the driving force in every happy activity in which he is employed. If at adolescence he is able to study and work towards a definite career, he is enabled to do this through the transformation of this same sexual energy. In the ordinary case the thing which prevents a man from working for his career is not intellectual defect and physical ill-health but emotional conflict, and the conflict centres on sexual problems. It helps us to get this matter in perspective if we realize that a boy of three unconsciously wants to be as potent as his father and envies his powers, or that a girl of that age wants to make a baby as her mother can. They have both to wait a long time, an interminable time, but the parent who knows and understands this will treat a child quite differently from one who does not. I do not mean that by talking of these things directly, or even by answering questions, the right results are achieved, but that a proper orientation to the child's play and behaviour, even when this is erotic, and the recognition of the value of such beginnings assists the child in his subsequent development.

Any serious difficulty in connection with the development of the child's sexuality will be manifested in several ways, such as prolonged moodiness and unhappiness, inhibition in games and learning, prolonged defiance, or on the other hand, passive goodness, obedience and docility. All such disturbances are referable ultimately to sexual fantasies and to a hitch in the effective use of sexual energy. Another problem inseparable from this is that of prolonged surreptitious forms of bodily gratifications. Adequate bodily gratifications of a sensuous kind are themselves a necessity and parents who recognize this necessity meet it by the provision of games, exercise, rhythmic movements, dancing, music, etc. Added to this, any normal child will indulge in investigation of itself and obtain gratification by masturbatory activities occasionally. It is the guilt attached to these actions and prolongation of them (causing lack of interest in social activities) which are the problems that call for expert help. Knowledge on the parents' part is a great help in producing a non-anxious attitude. If a child is punished or threatened whenever it is discovered in sexual activities its current difficulties are enormously increased, and inhibitory forces are set going which may prevent subsequent development. One must not expect, for instance, that a child who is punished and threatened for playing with five fingers on its body (from which it is getting a pleasurable sensation) is going later on to be an expert with its fingers on a piano. When a pleasure has been forbidden and cut off from its dynamic root, a vital function is threatened.

A child who thrusts its sexuality forward is in fact a worried child, more under the influence of anxiety than the average : its sexual urge as such may not be precocious but its sexual expression is being used to master its nervous fears. Let me illustrate : a child whose suckling has been marked by anxiety, or for whom there has been much frustration, will be difficult to wean, thumb sucking will probably be excessive ; if this is interfered with drastically one may be sure that masturbatory methods of getting gratifications will follow and will be attended with guilt and anxiety. More frustration than can be borne evokes aggression, which is expressed in the child's mind by a fantasy in which those who provoke him are slain. These fantasies lead to a premature arousing of erotic activities, for abnormal manifestations of sexual activities are really attempts to deal with abnormal quantities of aggression. Harsh dealing with the sexual activities is no solution of the problem at all. The matter of importance is to deal with aggression that lies at the root of abnormal sexual development.

Can we plan for stability ?

All conscious planning is of secondary importance to the environment provided by the parents' own emotional responses, subjective bias and prejudices. Upon their ability to recognize these, and so control and modify their own anxieties, depends the success of any plan, however seemingly wise and rational in conscious intent; any consciously adopted plan for upbringing needs to be based upon the following fundamental considerations.

Every child has an individual tempo of growth and co-ordination, and to interfere with this is to hinder natural growth; to retard or accelerate it is equally harmful. The responsiveness of the child must not be provoked, and time must be given for him to master his environment. The environment should not be changed too frequently.

The freer from anxiety the suckling period and the more skilful the handling of anxiety attacks in this period, the better the foundation of the child's life.

All activity of a happy nature is itself the utilization of sexual power and the basis of sublimation, hence the parent must not be stern or repressive or use threats concerning any sexual activity, but should provide channels for the utilization of energy. This libidinal drive brings richness and fulfilment to existence.

The child's psychical entity must be respected and the fact recognized that it must pass through crises in his development towards stability. The child will need time to master these, to work his way out and assimilate experience. We should recognize that a child needs psychical help if too many psychical stimuli assail him at one time, so that he cannot adequately master them alone.

Parents should be able to recognize what constitutes a psychical trauma.

There is an order of psychical development; for instance, there is an age when it is normal for a child to be destructive. There is an age when continued destructiveness is abnormal and requires specific therapeutic help, and (what is just as important to know) if a child at certain ages is passively good and docile, he certainly needs help. The criterion of goodness and badness of behaviour should not be the parents' present convenience but the ultimate stability of the child's personality.

Lastly, the absolute reliability of the parental figures is the child's mainstay through all its own changing world. His great need in early years is that his own emotional adjustments should be made within a stable and secure environment, not a cast-iron and rigid one, but one in which there is an orderly life, dictated by unfailing love and implicit faith. This implicit faith is founded upon the fact that psychical health, no less than physical, depends upon attunement with universal laws which support and uphold all order and all life.

These are the dynamics of human behaviour and determine it. I have indicated how within the basic community, the home, the conscious planning of the parents, however seemingly wise and rational, if it has not been subjected to investigation in the light of their own subjective wishes, may fail to bring about the conscious goal they have in mind. I have indicated that conscious plans not only need this deeper personal scrutiny, but that they must be based upon a deeper insight into the mental growth of the child and be flexibly orientated to the individual need. Along such lines environmental changes within the home can make for the more successful upbringing of children. The extension of these fundamental principles in the course of time, so that they are the bases upon which national schemes of education may be built, will alone make those environmental changes in the social order which is the conscious goal of our social endeavour.

II. WEANING

BY MELANIE KLEIN

ONE of the most fundamental and far-reaching discoveries ever made in human history was Freud's finding that there exists an unconscious part of the mind and that the nucleus of this unconscious mind is developed in earliest infancy. Infantile feelings and fantasies leave, as it were, their imprints on the mind, imprints which do not fade away but get stored up, remain active, and exert a continuous and powerful influence on the emotional and intellectual life of the individual. The earliest feelings are experienced in connection with external and internal stimuli. The first gratification which the child derives from the external world is the satisfaction experienced in being fed. Analysis has shown that only one part of this satisfaction results from the alleviation of hunger and that another part, no less important, results from the pleasure which the baby experiences when his mouth is stimulated by sucking at his mother's breast. This gratification is an essential part of the child's sexuality, and is indeed its initial expression. Pleasure is experienced also when the warm stream of milk runs down the throat and fills the stomach.

The baby reacts to unpleasant stimuli, and to the frustration of his pleasure, with feelings of hatred and aggression. These feelings of hatred are directed towards the same object as are the pleasurable ones, namely, the breasts of the mother.

Analytic work has shown that babies of a few months of age certainly indulge in fantasy building. I believe that this is the most primitive mental activity and that fantasies are in the mind of the infant almost from birth. It would seem that every stimulus the child receives is immediately responded to by fantasies, the unpleasant stimuli, including mere frustration, by fantasies of an aggressive kind, the gratifying stimuli by those focusing on pleasure.

As I said before, the object of all these fantasies is, to begin with, the breast of the mother. It may seem curious that the tiny child's interest should be limited to a part of a person rather than to the whole, but one must bear in mind first of all that the child has an extremely undeveloped capacity for perception, physical and mental, at this stage, and then we must remember the all-important fact that the tiny child is only concerned with his immediate gratification or the lack of it; Freud called this the " pleasure-pain principle ". Thus the breast of the mother which gives gratification or denies it becomes, in the mind of the child, imbued with the characteristics of good and evil. Now, what one might call the " good " breasts become the prototype of what is felt throughout life to be good and beneficent, while the " bad " breasts stand for everything evil and persecuting. The reason for this can be explained by the fact that, when the child turns his hatred against the denying or " bad " breast, he attributes to the breast itself all his own active hatred against it—a process which is termed *projection*.

But there is another process of great importance going on at the same time, namely, that of *intro-jection*. By this is meant the mental activity in the child, by which, in his fantasy, he takes into himself everything which he perceives in the outside world. We know that at this stage the child receives his main satisfaction through his mouth, which therefore becomes the main channel through which the child takes in not only his food, but also, in his fantasy, the world outside him. Not only the mouth, but to a certain degree the whole body with all its senses and functions, performs this " taking in " process—for instance, the child breathes in, takes in through his eyes, his ears, through touch and so on. To begin with, the breast of the mother is the object of his constant desire, and therefore this is the first thing to be introjected. In fantasy the child sucks the breast into himself, chews it up and swallows it ; thus he feels that he has actually got it there, that he possesses the mother's breast within himself, in both its good and in its bad aspects.

The child's focusing on and attachment to a part of the person is characteristic of this early stage of development, and accounts in great measure for the fantastic and unrealistic nature of his relation to everything, for example, to parts of his own body, to people and to inanimate objects, all of which are at first of course only dimly perceived. The object

world of the child in the first two or three months
of its life could be described as consisting of
gratifying or of hostile and persecuting parts or
portions of the real world. At about this age he
begins to see his mother and others about him as
" whole people ", his realistic perception of her
(and them) coming gradually as he connects her
face looking down at him with the hands that
caress him and with the breast that satisfies him,
and the power to perceive " wholes " (once the
pleasure in " whole persons " is assured and he
has confidence in them) spreads to the external
world beyond the mother.

At this time other changes too are taking place in
the child. When the baby is a few weeks old, one
can observe that he begins definitely to enjoy
periods in his waking life ; judging by appearances,
there are times when he feels quite happy. It seems
that at about the age just mentioned localized overstrong stimuli diminish (in the beginning, for
instance, defæcation is often felt as unpleasant),
and a much better co-ordination begins to be
established in the exercise of the different bodily
functions. This leads not only to a better physical
but also to a better mental adaptation to external
and internal stimuli. One can surmise that stimuli
which at first were felt as painful, no longer are so
and some of them have even become pleasant. The
fact that lack of stimuli can now be felt as an enjoyment in itself, indicates that he is no longer so
much swayed by painful feelings, caused by unpleasant stimuli, or so avid for pleasurable ones
in connection with the immediate and full gratifica-

tion given by feeding; his better adaptation towards stimuli renders the necessity for immediate and strong gratification less urgent.[1]

I have referred to the early fantasies and fears of persecution in connection with the hostile breasts, and I have explained how they are connected with the fantastic object-relationship of the tiny child. The child's earliest experiences of painful external and internal stimuli provide a basis for fantasies about hostile external and internal objects, and they contribute largely to the building up of such fantasies.[2]

In the earliest stage of mental development every unpleasant stimulus is apparently related in the baby's fantasy to the " hostile " or denying breasts, every pleasant stimulus on the other hand to the " good ", gratifying breasts. It seems that here we have two circles, the one benevolent and the other vicious, both of which are based on the interplay of external or environmental and internal psychical factors; thus any lessening of the amount or intensity of painful stimuli or any increase in the capacity to adjust to them should help to diminish the strength of fantasies of a frightening nature, and a decrease of frightening fantasies in its turn enables the child to take steps towards a better adaptation to reality, and this helps to diminish the frightening fantasies.

[1] In this connection I am reminded of a comment made recently by Dr. Edward Glover; he pointed out that the abrupt change between very painful and very pleasurable sensations might be felt as painful in itself.

[2] Dr. Susan Isaacs emphasized the importance of this point in a paper to the British Psycho-Analytical Society (January, 1934).

It is important for the proper development of the mind that the child should come under the influence of the benevolent circle I have just outlined ; when this happens he is greatly assisted in forming an image of his mother as a person ; this growing perception of the mother as a whole implies not only very important changes in his intellectual, but also in his emotional development.

I have already mentioned that fantasies and feelings of an aggressive and of a gratifying, erotic nature, which are to a large extent fused together (a fusion which is called sadism), play a dominant part in the child's early life. They are first of all focused on the breasts of his mother, but gradually extend to her whole body. Greedy, erotic and destructive fantasies and feelings have for their object the inside of the mother's body. In his imagination the child attacks it, robbing it of everything it contains and eating it up.

At first the destructive fantasies are more of a sucking nature. Something of this is shown in the powerful way with which some children will suck, even when milk is plentiful. The nearer the child comes to the time of cutting teeth, the more the fantasies take on the nature of biting, tearing, chewing up and thus destroying their object. Many mothers find that long before the child cuts his teeth these biting tendencies show themselves. Analytic experience has proved that these tendencies go along with fantasies of a definitely cannibalistic nature. The destructive quality of all these sadistic fantasies and feelings, as we find from the analysis of small children, is in full swing when the child begins to perceive his mother as a whole person.

At the same time he now experiences a change in his emotional attitude towards the mother. The child's pleasurable attachment to the breast develops into feelings towards her as a person. Thus feelings both of a destructive and of a loving nature are experienced towards one and the same person and this gives rise to deep and disturbing conflicts in the child's mind.

It is, in my view, very important for the child's future that he should be able to progress from the early fears of persecution and a fantastic object-relationship to the relation to the mother as a whole person and a loving being. When, however, he succeeds in doing this, feelings of guilt arise in connection with the child's own destructive impulses, which he now fears to be a danger to his loved object. The fact that at this stage of development the child is unable to control his sadism, as it wells up at any frustration, still further aggravates the conflict and his concern for the loved one. Again it is very important that the child should deal satisfactorily with these conflicting feelings—love, hatred and guilt—which are aroused in this new situation. If the conflicts prove unbearable the child cannot establish a happy relationship with his mother, and the way lies open for many failures in subsequent development. I wish especially to mention states of undue or abnormal depression which, in my view, have their deepest source in the failure to deal satisfactorily with these early conflicts.

But let us now consider what happens when the feelings of guilt and fear of the death of his mother (which is dreaded as a result of his unconscious wishes for her death) are dealt with adequately. These feelings have, I think, far-reaching effects on the child's future mental well-being, his capacity for love and his social development. From them springs *the desire to restore*, which expresses itself in numerous fantasies of saving her and making all kinds of reparation. These tendencies to make reparation I have found in the analysis of small children to be the driving forces in all constructive activities and interests, and for social development. We find them at work in the first play-activities and at the basis of the child's satisfaction in his achievements, even those of the most simple kind for example, in putting one brick on top of another, or making a brick stand upright after it had been knocked down—all this is partly derived from the unconscious fantasy of making some kind of restoration to some person or several persons whom he has injured in fantasy. But more than this, even the much earlier achievements of the baby, such as playing with his fingers, finding something which had rolled aside, standing up and all sorts of voluntary movements—these too, I believe, are connected with fantasies in which the reparation element is already present.

The analysis of quite small children—in recent years children of even between one and two years have been analysed—show that babies of a few months connect their fæces and urine with fantasies in which these materials are regarded as presents.

Not only are they presents, and as such are indications of love towards their mother or nurse, but they are also regarded as being able to effect a restoration. On the other hand, when the destructive feelings are dominant the baby will in his fantasy defæcate and urinate in anger and hatred, and use his excrements as hostile agents. Thus the excrements produced with friendly feelings are, in fantasy, used as a means of making good the injuries inflicted also by the agency of fæces and urine in moments of anger.

It is impossible within the scope of this paper to deal adequately with the connection between aggressive fantasies, fears, feelings of guilt and the wish to make reparation; nevertheless, I have touched on this topic because I wanted to indicate that aggressive feelings, which lead to so much disturbance in the child's mentality, are at the same time of the highest value for his development.

I have already mentioned that the child mentally takes into himself—introjects—the outside world as far as he can perceive it. First he introjects the good and bad breasts, but gradually it is the whole mother (again conceived as a good and bad mother) which he takes into himself. Along with this the father and the other people in the child's surroundings are taken in as well, to begin with in a lesser degree but in the same manner as the relation to the mother; these figures grow in importance and acquire independence in the child's mind as time goes on. If the child succeeds in establishing within himself a kind and helpful mother, this internalized mother will prove a most beneficial influence throughout his whole life. Though this influence will normally change in character with the development of the mind, it is comparable with the vitally important place that the real mother has in the tiny child's very existence. I do not mean that the "internalized" good parents will consciously be felt as such (even in the small child the feeling of possessing them inside is deeply unconscious), they are not felt consciously to be there, but rather as something within the personality having the nature of kindness and wisdom; this leads to confidence and trust in oneself and helps to combat and overcome the feelings of fear of having bad figures within one and of being governed by one's own uncontrollable hatred; and furthermore, this leads to trust in people in the outside world beyond the family circle.

As I have pointed out above, the child feels any frustration very acutely; though some progress towards adaptation to reality is normally going on all the time, the child's emotional life seems dominated by the cycle of gratification and frustration; but the feelings of frustration are of a very complicated nature. Dr. Ernest Jones found that frustration is always felt as deprivation, if the child cannot obtain the desired thing, he feels that it is being withheld by the nasty mother, who has power over him.

Coming to our main problem, we find that the child feels, when the breast is wanted but is not there, as if it were lost for ever; since the conception of the breast extends to that of the mother, the feelings of having lost the breast lead to the fear of having lost the loved mother entirely, and this means not only the real mother, but also the good mother within. In my experience this fear of the total loss of the good object (internalized and external) is interwoven with feelings of guilt at having destroyed her (eaten her up), and then the child feels that her loss is a punishment for his dreadful deed; thus the most distressing and conflicting feelings become associated with frustration, and it is these which make the pain of what seems like a simple thwarting so poignant. The actual experience of weaning greatly reinforces these painful feelings or tends to substantiate these fears; but in so far as the baby never has uninterrupted possession of the breast, and over and over again is in the state of lacking it, one could say that, in a sense, he is in a constant state of being weaned or at least in a state leading up to weaning. Nevertheless, the crucial point is reached at the actual weaning when the loss is complete and the breast or bottle is gone irrevocably.

I might quote from my experience a case in which the feelings connected with this loss were very clearly shown. Rita, aged two years and nine months when she came for analysis, was a very neurotic child with fears of all kinds, and most difficult to bring up; her quite unchildlike depressions and feelings of guilt were very striking. She was very much tied to her mother, displaying at times an exaggerated love and at others antagonism. She was, at the time she came to me, still having one bottle at night-time and the mother told me that she had had to continue this, since she had found that the child showed too much distress when she attempted to stop giving it to her. Rita's weaning had been very difficult. She had been breast fed for a few months, had then been given bottles which at first she did not want to accept, then she got used to them, and displayed again great difficulties when the bottles were replaced by ordinary food. When, during her analysis with me, she was weaned from this last bottle, she fell into a state of despair. She lost her appetite, refused food, clung more than ever to her mother, asking her constantly whether she loved her, if she had been naughty, and so on. It could not have been a question of food in itself, as the milk was only a part of her diet, and moreover the same amount of milk was given to her, but out of a glass. I had advised the mother to give Rita the milk herself, adding a biscuit or two, and sitting at her bedside or taking her on her lap. But the child did not want to have the milk. Her analysis revealed that her despair was due to her anxiety of her mother's death or to the fear of her mother punishing her cruelly for her badness. What she felt as " badness " actually was her unconscious wishes for her mother's death both in the present and in the past. She was overwhelmed by anxiety of having destroyed, and especially of having eaten up her mother, and the loss of the bottle was felt as the confirmation that she had done so. Even looking at her mother did not disprove these fears until they were resolved by analysis. In this case the early fears of persecution had not been sufficiently overcome, and the personal relation to the mother had never been well established. This failure was on the one hand due to the child's inability to deal with her overstrong conflicts, on the other hand—and this again becomes part of the internal conflict—to the actual conduct of her mother who was a highly neurotic person.

It is evident that a good human relationship between the child and his mother at the time when these basic conflicts set in and are largely worked through is of the highest value. We must remember that at the critical time of weaning the child, as it were, loses his " good " object, that is, he loses what he loves most. Anything which makes the loss of an external good object less painful, and diminishes the fear of being punished, will help the child to preserve the belief in his good object within. At the same time it will prepare the way for the child to keep up, in spite of the frustration, a happy relation to his real mother and to establish pleasurable relations with people other than his parents. Then he will succeed in obtaining satisfactions, which will replace the all-important one which he is just about to lose.

Now, what can we do to help the child in this difficult task ? The preparations for this task start at birth. From the very beginning the mother must do everything she can to help the child to establish a happy relationship with her. So often we find that the mother does everything in her power for the child's physical condition ; she concentrates on this as if the child were a material thing which needs constant upkeep, like a valuable machine rather than a human being. This is the attitude of many pediatricians who are mostly concerned with the physical development of the child, and are only interested in his emotional reactions in so far as they indicate something about his physical or intellectual state. Mothers often do not realize that a tiny baby is already a human being whose emotional development is of highest importance.

A good contact between mother and child may be jeopardized at the first or the first few feeds by the fact that the mother does not know how to induce the baby to take the nipple; if, for example, instead of dealing patiently with the difficulties as they arise, the nipple is pushed rather roughly into the baby's mouth, he may fail to develop a strong attachment to the nipple and to the breast, and become a difficult feeder. On the other hand, one can observe how babies who show this initial difficulty develop under patient assistance into quite as good feeders as those who have no initial difficulty at all.[1]

There are many other occasions than just at the breast when the baby will feel and unconsciously record his mother's love, patience and understanding —or the contrary. As I have already pointed out, the earliest feelings are experienced in connection with internal and external stimuli—pleasant or unpleasant—and are associated with fantasies. The way in which the baby is handled even from the time of delivery from the womb is bound to leave impressions on his mind.

[1] I have to thank Dr. D. Winnicott for many illuminating details on this subject.

Though the infant in the earliest stage of his development cannot yet relate the pleasant feelings, which the care and patience of the mother rouse in him, to her as a "whole person", it is of vital importance that these pleasurable feelings and the sense of trust should be experienced. Everything which makes the baby feel that it is surrounded with friendly objects, though these are, to begin with, conceived of, for the most part, as "good breasts", prepares the ground for and contributes to the building up of a happy relation to the mother and later on to other people around him.

A balance must be kept between physical and psychical necessities. The regularity of feeding has proved to be of great value for the baby's physical well-being, and this again influences the psychical development; but there are many children who, in the early days at any rate, cannot easily sustain breaks of too long duration between the feeds; in these cases it is better not to keep rigidly to rules, and to feed the baby every three hours or even under this, and, if necessary, to give a sip of dill-water or sugar water in between times.

I think the use of the comforter is helpful. It is true that it has a disadvantage—not of a hygienic nature, for that can be overcome—the psychological disadvantage is the disappointment for the baby, when in sucking he does not receive the desired milk, but at any rate he has the partial gratification in being able to suck. If he is not allowed the comforter he will probably all the more suck his fingers; as the use of the comforter can be better regulated than the sucking of the fingers, the baby can better be weaned from the comforter. One might begin the weaning gradually, e.g., to give it only before the child settles down to sleep, or if he is not quite well, and so on.

As regards the question of weaning from thumb-sucking, Dr. Middlemore (Chapter IV) expresses the opinion that on the whole the child should not be weaned from sucking his thumb. There is something to be said in favour of this view. Frustrations which can be avoided should not be inflicted on the child. Furthermore, there is the fact to be considered that overstrong frustrations of the mouth may lead to an intensified need for compensatory genital pleasure, for example, compulsive masturbation, and that some of the intrinsic frustrations experienced at the mouth are carried over to the genital.

But there are other aspects to be considered as well. In unbridled sucking of the thumb or the comforter there is a danger of overstrong mouth-fixation ; (I mean by this that the libido is hindered in its natural movement from the mouth to the genital), while mild frustration of the mouth would have the desirable effect of distributing the sensual urges.

Continual sucking may act inhibitively upon speech development. Furthermore, the sucking of the thumbs, if excessive, has this disadvantage : the child often hurts himself, and then he not only experiences physical pain, but the connection between the pleasure in sucking and the pain in his fingers is psychologically disadvantageous.

With regard to masturbation I should say definitely that it ought not to be interfered with, the child should be left to deal with this in his own way.[1] With regard to the thumb-sucking, I should say that it can in many cases be replaced without pressure partly and gradually with other oral gratifications, such as sweets, fruit and specially favoured foods. These one should provide for the child *ad libitum*, while at the same time, with the help of the comforter, one softens the process of weaning.

Another point I want to stress is the mistake of attempting too early to get the child used to habits of cleanliness in regard to his excretory functions. Some mothers are proud of having achieved this task very early, but they do not realize the bad psychological effects to which it may give rise. I don't mean to say that there is any harm in holding the baby from time to time over a chamber and

[1] If the masturbation is done obtrusively or excessively—and the same applies to prolonged and excessively hard thumb-sucking—one may find that something is wrong with the child's relation to his environment. For instance, he may feel afraid of his nurse without this ever coming to the knowledge of his parents. He may feel unhappy at school because he feels backward or because he is on bad terms with a certain teacher or afraid of another child. In analyses one discovers that such things can account for an increased strain on the child's mind which finds relief in increased and compulsive sensual gratification. Naturally, the removal of external factors will not always alleviate the strain, but with such children a reprimand for the excessive masturbation can only add to the underlying difficulties. When these are so great, they can be removed only by a psychological treatment.

47

thus begin to accustom him gently to it. The point in question is that the mother ought not to be over-anxious, and ought not to try to prevent the child from ever dirtying or wetting himself. The baby senses this attitude towards his excrements and feels disturbed by it, for he takes a strong sexual pleasure in his excretory functions and he likes his excrements as a part and product of his own body. On the other hand, as I pointed out before, he feels that his fæces and urine are hostile agents when he defæcates and urinates with angry feelings. If the mother anxiously tries to prevent him from getting in contact with them altogether, the baby feels this behaviour as a confirmation that his excrements are evil and hostile agents of which the mother is afraid : her anxiety increases his. This attitude to his own excrements is psychologically detrimental, and plays a great part in many neuroses.

Of course I do not mean to say that the baby ought to be allowed to lie dirty indefinitely ; what to my mind should be avoided is making his cleanliness a matter of such importance, because then the child senses how anxious the mother is over it. The whole thing should be taken easily and signs of disgust or disapproval while cleaning the baby should be avoided. I think that a *systematic* training in cleanliness is better postponed until after weaning. This training is certainly a considerable strain both mentally and physically on the baby and one that ought not to be imposed on him while he is coping with the difficulties of weaning. Even later on this training should not be carried out with any strictness, as Dr. Isaacs will show in her chapter on " Habit ".

It is a great asset for the future relationship between mother and child if the mother not only feeds but nurses her baby as well. If circumstances prevent her from doing so she may still be able to establish a strong bond between herself and her baby, if she has insight into the baby's mentality.

The baby can enjoy his mother's presence in so many ways. He will often have a little play with her breast after feeding, he will take pleasure in her looking at him, smiling at him, playing with him and talking to him long before he understands the meaning of words. He will get to know and to like her voice, and her singing to him may remain a pleasurable and stimulating memory in his unconscious. Soothing him in this way, how often she can avert tension and avoid an unhappy state of mind, and thus put him to sleep instead of letting him fall asleep exhausted with crying!

A really happy relationship between mother and child can be established only when nursing and feeding the baby is not a matter of duty but a real pleasure to the mother. If she can enjoy it thoroughly, her pleasure will be unconsciously realized by the child, and this reciprocal happiness will lead to a full emotional understanding between mother and child.

But there is another side to the picture. The mother must realize that the baby is not actually her possession, and that, though he is so small and utterly dependent on her help, he is a separate entity and ought to be treated as an individual human being; she must not tie him too much to herself, but assist him to grow up to independence. The earlier she can take up this attitude the better; she will thus not only help the child, but preserve herself from future disappointment.

The child's development ought not to be unduly interfered with. It is one thing to watch with enjoyment and understanding his mental and physical growth, and another thing to try to accelerate it. The baby ought to be left to grow quietly in his own way. As Ella Sharpe has mentioned in the preceding chapter, the desire to impose a rate of growth upon the child, to make it fit into a prearranged plan, is detrimental to the child and to his relationship to the mother. Her desire to speed on progress is often due to anxiety, which is one of the main sources of disturbance in the mother-child relationship.

There is another matter in which the mother's attitude is of highest importance, and that is in regard to the sexual development of the child, that is, his experiences of bodily sexual sensations and the accompanying desires and feelings. It is not yet generally realized that the infant from birth onwards has strong sexual feelings, which, to begin with, manifest themselves through the pleasure experienced in his mouth activities and excretory functions, but which very soon get connected with the genitals as well (masturbation); nor is it generally and sufficiently realized that these sexual feelings are essential for the proper development of the child, and that his personality and character, as well as a satisfactory adult sexuality, depend on his sexuality being established in child-hood.

I have already pointed out that one should not interfere with the child's masturbation, nor exert pressure in weaning him from thumb-sucking, and that one should be understanding about the pleasure he takes in his excretory functions and his excreta. But that alone is not sufficient. The mother must have a really friendly attitude towards these mani-festations of his sexuality. So often she is apt to show disgust, harshness or scorn which is both humiliating and detrimental to the child. Since all his erotic trends are directed first and foremost towards his mother and father, their reactions will influence his whole development in these matters. On the other hand, there is also the question of too great indulgence to be considered. Though the child's sexuality is not to be interfered with, the mother might have to restrain him—of course in a friendly way—if he should attempt to take too much liberty with her person. Neither must the mother allow herself to become involved in his sexuality. A really friendly acceptance of sexuality in her child constitutes the limit of her rôle. Her own erotic needs must be well controlled where he is concerned. She must not become passionately excited by any of her activities in tending the child. When washing, drying or powdering him restraint is necessary, particularly in connection with the genital regions. The mother's lack of self-control may easily be felt by the child as a seduction, and this would set up undue complications in his development. Yet the child should by no means be deprived of love. The mother certainly can and ought to kiss and caress him and take him on her lap, all of which he needs and is only to his good.

This leads me to another important point. It is essential that the baby should not sleep in his parents' bedroom and be present during sexual intercourse. People often think that this is not harmful for the baby, because, for one thing, they do not realize that his sexual feelings, his aggression and fears get too much stirred through such an experience, and they further ignore the fact that the baby takes in unconsciously what he seems unable to grasp intellectually. Often, when the parents think the baby is asleep, he is awake or half awake, and even when he seems to be asleep he is able to sense what is going on around him. Though everything is perceived only in a dim way, a vivid, but distorted memory remains active in his unconscious mind, and has harmful effects on his development. Especially bad is the effect when this experience coincides with others which also put a strain on the child, for example, an illness, an operation or—to come back to the topic of my chapter—the weaning.

I should like to say now a few words about the actual process of the weaning from the breast. It seems to me of great importance to do this slowly and gently. If the baby is to be completely weaned, let us say, at eight or nine months—which seems the right age—at about five or six months, for one breast-feeding a day a bottle should be substituted, and every subsequent month another bottle should take the place of a breast-feeding. At the same time other suitable food should be introduced, and when the child has got used to this, one can begin to wean him from the bottle, which then will be replaced partly by other food and partly by milk drunk out of a glass. The weaning will be greatly facilitated if patience and gentleness are exercised in accustoming the child to new food. The child ought not to be made to eat more than he wants, or to eat food he dislikes—on the contrary, he should be provided with the food he likes in plenty—nor should table manners play any part at this period.

So far I have said nothing about upbringing where the baby is not breast fed. I hope I have made clear the great psychological importance of the mother feeding her child ; let us now consider the eventuality of the mother's being unable to do this.

The bottle is a substitute for the mother's breast, for it allows the baby to have the pleasure of sucking and thus to establish to a certain degree the breast-mother relationship in connection with the bottle given by the mother or nurse.

Experience shows that often children who have not been breast fed develop quite well.[1] Still, in analysis one will always discover in such people a deep longing for the breast which has never been fulfilled, and though the breast-mother relationship

[1] More than this, even children who have gone through very difficult experiences in this early period, such as illnesses, sudden weaning or an operation, often develop quite satisfactorily, though such experiences are always in one way or another a handicap and should, of course, if possible be avoided.

has been established to a certain degree, it makes all the difference to the psychic development that the earliest and fundamental gratification has been obtained from a substitute, instead of from the real thing which was desired. One may say that although children can develop well without being breast fed, the development would have been different and better in one way or another had they had a successful breast-feeding. On the other hand, I infer from my experience that children whose development goes wrong, even though they have been breast fed, would have been more ill without it.

To summarize: successful breast-feeding is always an important asset for development; some children, though they have missed this fundamentally favourable influence, develop very well without it.

In this chapter I have discussed the methods which might help to make the sucking period and the weaning successful; I am now in the rather difficult position of having to tell you that what may seem to be a success is not necessarily a complete one. Although some children appear to have gone through the weaning quite well and even for some time progress satisfactorily, deep down they have been unable to deal with the difficulties arising out of this situation; only an outward adaptation has taken place. This outward adaptation results from the child's urge to please those around him, upon whom he is so dependent, and from his desire to be on good terms with them. This drive in the child manifests itself to a certain degree even as early as in the weaning period; I believe that babies have altogether much more intellectual capacity than is assumed. There is another important reason for this mainly outward adaptation, namely, that it serves as an escape from the deep inner conflicts which the child is unable to deal with. In other cases, there are more obvious signs of the failure of true adaptation; for instance, in many character defects, such as jealousy, greed and resentfulness. In this connection I would mention Dr. Karl Abraham's work on the relation between early difficulties and the formation of character.

We all know people who go about in life with constant grievances. For instance, they resent even the bad weather as a thing especially inflicted upon them by a hostile fate. Again, there are others who turn away from every gratification if it does not come immediately when it is wanted; in the words of the popular song of a few years ago, " I want what I want when I want it, or I don't want it at all."

I have endeavoured to show you that frustration is so difficult for the infant to bear because of the deep inner conflicts which are connected with it. A really successful weaning implies that the baby has not only got used to new food, but that it has actually made the first and fundamental steps towards dealing with its inner conflicts and fears, and that it is thus finding adjustment to frustration in its true sense.

If this adjustment has been made, then weaning in the obsolete sense of the word can here be applied. I understand that in old English the word weaning was used not only in the sense of "weaning from" but also of "weaning to." Applying these two senses of the word, we may say that when real adaptation to frustration has taken place, the individual is weaned not only from his mother's breasts, but towards substitutes—towards all those sources of gratification and satisfaction which are needed for building up a full, rich and happy life.

NOTE: A postscript to this paper, written in January 1952, appears on page 233.

III. THE USES OF SENSUALITY

BY MERELL P. MIDDLEMORE, M.D.

BEFORE I say anything about the use of sensuality I must define the word, so that when I speak of it we shall be thinking about the same thing.

I take sensuality to be the enjoyment of any bodily feeling; and the problem before us is whether, by judicious planning, we can help the child, as he becomes aware of his various feelings, still to remain free from the sense of guilt and fear which is so often associated with bodily pleasure. If this can be done, sensuality will prove to be a strong foundation for his favourable psychical development.

You may, of course, object to my definition of sensuality and say that bodily feelings which are shocking at first experience may later prove to be delightful. " At what moment," you will ask, " does a cold shower begin to give sensual pleasure ? " Not at the first application to be sure, but later it may give a great deal. Now as far as we know at present, many of the sensations which the young child first experiences are like the cold shower—they have to be repeated again and again before they are enjoyed. Thus Charlotte Bühler, the Austrian psychologist, after making a series of observations on infants, came

57

to a startling conclusion.[1] She found that from birth to the third month of life the baby makes more gestures of distress than he does of pleasure —that he spends more of his waking time crying or grimacing than contented, and that speaking in a general way he actually dislikes being touched and moved, seeing light or hearing voices.

Why he dislikes disturbances which are apparently quite pleasant isn't so clear. We can guess that all ordinary forms of stimulation are too strong for an organism which, until the day of birth, has seen no light at all and felt no direct touch on its body. We know that the new-born baby carries on the essential bodily processes of breathing, circulation and nutrition, all of which give rise to strong internal feeling, but that he is pitifully defenceless in face of external stimulation. He cannot even turn his head away from a bright light to begin with, and the only co-ordinated response which brings him into touch with other people is the act of sucking. For the rest he must gradually learn to react appropriately so as to avoid stimulation or to discharge as quickly as he can whatever tension follows it. I think of tension in the infant as a bodily state in which stimulation irks him— light is dazzling instead of being agreeable, a smell is overpowering and emotions are too strong to arouse pleasant feelings only. It corresponds with the adult state of being " on edge ", though in this case emphasis is laid on the mental rather than the physical condition.

Why some movements successfully relieve ten-

[1] Charlotte Bühler, *The First Year of Life*, 1930,

sion and others fail I cannot say ; though I can point out that those which bring most pleasurable relief are not only co-ordinated movements but rhythmic ones. And here you will remember that a new-born child can practise only one well-co-ordinated reaction—his sucking ; so that he is ill-equipped to deal with any variety of external stimulus.

Now contrast this early stage with a later one when he is, say, six months old. What is the difference between them ? At birth stimulation was a menace ; at six months old, when the child has developed all sorts of co-ordinated responses to it, he positively enjoys it.

Another aspect of the child's changing response to sensual stimulation calls for attention. Although the mouth never has a monopoly of feeling and action, at birth it is the most acutely feeling and efficiently acting organ of the body, and the infant's behaviour is orientated round mouth sensation. As the days pass, the baby becomes increasingly aware of other sensations, and he distributes among them the interest which he used to concentrate on the mouth. After a period of diffused interest a reorientation takes place in his behaviour, and, towards the end of his first year, anal function comes to dominate his fantasy as mouth function did before. External events help to bring about the change, for about this time the baby loses the delightful and repeated contact of mouth with nipple, and in most cases the mother, who no longer lets him have the nipple, begins to show more concern with his bowel actions.

We have good reason to believe that bowel sensations are strongly felt from the first week of life onwards and thus influence the child's early mental development, and that the same thing is true of genital feeling. But each of these feelings seems to exert its maximum influence on the child at a different stage in his life—anal feelings reach a climax in the later months of his first year, genital feelings in the later months of his second year. We must not assume, however, that anal sensation is most intense when the child is a year old and genital feeling when he is between two and three; for we cannot compare the strength of sensation as it is felt by the infant in the early days of life, and later, at the period of anal or genital primacy. So that I would rather say that the child's fantasy is likely to be occupied chiefly with anal and genital sensation respectively at the times I have indicated, though never to the exclusion of other bodily feelings ; for instance, mouth-pleasure will not fail during the months in which anal fantasy predominates.[1]

While we are considering in a general way the relation between sensation and fantasy I should like to compare the feelings which belong to the mouth, anus and genitals with those peculiar to the muscles,

[1] The classical studies on the sequence of sensation and fantasy are as follows : Sigm. Freud, *Drei Abhandlungen zur Sexualtheorie* (Wiem, 1905) ; Karl Abraham, " A Short Study of the Development of the Libido," 1924, in *Selected Papers of Karl Abraham* (London, 1927) ; Ernest Jones, " Hate and Anal Erotism in the Obsessional Neurosis," 1913, in *Papers on Psycho-Analysis*, 3rd edn. (London, 1923) ; " The Phallic Phase," *International Journal of Psycho-Analysis*, 1933, vol. xiv.

the respiratory tract, etc. Why are the former triad given pride of place when we estimate the influence exerted by sensation on psychical development ?

It is not enough to say that oral, anal and genital feelings are more acute than other bodily sensations, though this may well be true. Perhaps it is just as important that each of them is concentrated on a small area of mucous membrane, and that the mucous membrane concerned in each case surrounds an orifice of the body. The concentration of sensation in a small area allows a swift discharge of tension to follow by direct stimulation of one point. The situation of the sensitive area at a body orifice ensures that its stimulation shall give rise to fantasies about the material which passes over it on the way in or out of the body ; and when the fantasy is concerned with the child doing things to other people, he pictures himself breaking into them by the same ports of entry which are so sensitive in his own body.[1]

In this summary description of the development of the child's response to body sensation I have pointed out that enjoyment of bodily feeling steadily increases during the first months of life ; that there is first a selective interest and a pleasure in mouth sensation—an interest which passes from the mouth to the anus and genitals as the child grows older ; that every sensation has its psychic accompaniment of fantasy.

I want now to consider in detail three different

[1] Melanie Klein, *The Psycho-Analysis of Children*, London, 1932.

types of sensual experience : first, the sensuality of a single, independent sense area, and as an example we will take the mouth area ; next, the sensuality characterized by co-ordination of one sense area with another, for instance, the co-ordination of the muscle and tactile sense of the hand with sight and hearing ; finally, that sensuality which is derived partly from local genital feeling, and partly from a general reaction of the whole body to the stimulus of contact with people. In each case I hope to find out what immediate use sensuality has in the development of the young child.

Most regular of all exploitations of sensuality is the sucking of comforters and thumbs ; and everyone knows its immediate use to the baby—it relieves his tension by making bodily feeling enjoyable. He is teething, say, with pain in his gums, and when he grinds them on the comforter, he transmutes the pain into something more like excitement. Or when tension is general and the pain far removed from the mouth, sucking brings along pleasant feelings which can compete with the painful ones and come to occupy more and more of his attention. There is also an agreeable degree of tension that makes the baby suck gaily and feel at his best.

I would say at a venture about the pleasant feelings attendant on sucking that most of the satisfaction comes from the rhythmic movement of tongue, lips and jaws ; but the touch firmly made by the whole mouth on the thumb inside it can give pleasure too, so can a nice taste on the tongue and a gentle flow of saliva. All these things are appreciated by the infant's mouth. And what a highly specialized mouth it is! It somehow dominates the face and gropes after anything that comes near it ; while the inside of the lips are extraordinarily cushiony and sensitive, ready to enjoy the contacts of sucking as much as they can be enjoyed. So much for the physiological act of sucking.

We have also to consider its psychological accompaniments and its effect on the child's whole body and mind. To begin with, I suppose that the rhythmic movements and the feel of the small thumb lying inside the mouth conjure up memories of ardent or peaceful times which the baby spent sucking at the breast and of the fantasies he had meanwhile. If these memories and fantasies are happy ones they will give him pleasure later as he sucks his thumb, and his body will comfortably relax. But quite apart from any formal memory the whole business of sucking has on it the hallmark of familiarity—a body memory, one might call it—for the movements have been made and have given pleasure a thousand times before. I imagine also that it is partly the skill of the movements and their accustomed mastery over the thumb that make sucking so satisfactory to the child.

I remember a case which well illustrates the use of sucking as a familiar movement and a masterful one. . Once I watched a ten-months' baby who was in great pain when he was admitted to hospital, and during the hours he had to wait for operation he continually sucked his thumb. There was no delightful memory of feeding in this sucking ; it was done in a mood of frenzy. And his fantasy must have been a furious one, for besides sucking his thumb the baby began to bite it until it bled. Still he would not let it go for a moment and I gave up an attempt to rescue it because he grew desperate when he couldn't bite. I suppose that at the first niggling pain he stuck his thumb into his mouth because by all the rules of the game it ought to have comforted him when he was in the grip of colic; it ought to have distracted his troubled mind or set up a soothing rhythm in his body. But by the time I saw him he hoped for no such thing. He may have comforted himself by working his jaws in a familiar way, but the essential feature of the mouth movements was their attack on the thumb and their endeavour to hurt it as much as ever the colic hurt. And to me the significance of the whole incident lay in the fact that the baby broke into bitter crying directly I prevented him from biting himself.

Summarize the case: the baby could keep calm for just as long as he strongly stimulated the combined areas of thumb and mouth, and he maintained this calm in face of heavy odds and great pain. There is something to be learned from his story; for one thing, he could not deal with his misery except by using very fierce sensual stimulation—sucking was not enough to relieve his tension, he must bite. Let us immediately concede that he enjoyed biting, and that the combination of biting and pain set up some kind of psychic equilibrium in which he could most easily manage to live during his hours of distress; that is to say, he used his mouth sensuality and the pain in his thumb to maintain a balance of pleasure for his whole body; a real pleasure—for he burst into tears when it was taken away. And this is the fundamental use of all sensuality, whether the desired feeling comes from the mouth or the muscles, the anus or the genitals. But many of us lose sight of the urgent need to maintain a pleasure-balance in life when we think of conventional forms of sensuality which are simply pleasant in quality and are used in situations which do not subject the body to any special strain.

I would have you note at this point that by no amount of thought could I have guessed that a baby suffering from intussusception [1] would find his best emotional relief in thumb-biting. And while I have told you about a child who chose to bite when he was in trouble and when another would have screamed, you will realize that a third infant might have kicked and struck at me as if he struck the pain, and a fourth might have cuddled in my arms for comfort. For each child early develops his own bodily pleasures and his own ways of escape from tension, and this without our planning. All we can do is to see that he is not needlessly frustrated in the discharge of his instinctual drives.

Consider, for instance, the problem of genital feeling. It comes to the baby in due course, and just as tension set up by mouth feeling is relieved by sucking, so genital tension is relieved by mastur-

[1] A painful and dangerous abdominal condition with colic as an outstanding symptom.

bation. It is a normal activity of the young child, an important one also, for it discharges general tension so that body and mind are left at ease to work at their best, the body to make its various endeavours, the mind to take up new psychic impressions and comfortably to set them in order.

This sounds like an ideal state of affairs, and from it we must turn to practical aspects of the subject. What is the parent to do about thumb-sucking and masturbation? Can these gratifications do the child any harm? We know how often the young baby sucks his thumb or his toys when he is excited and lively, and it seems to me that when he is unhappy the remedy most appropriate to his age is mouth pleasure. I have reminded you how highly specialized is the mouth of the suckling and it doesn't worry me how much he uses it. He must get due release from tension. I go further and strongly deprecate the use of woolly gloves at night or any device which is meant to make his sucking less useful. In the same way I would let a little child masturbate if he wants to, simply making sure that he has enough diverting things to play with and that he is encouraged to scramble about the house and garden seeking his own adventures. Excessive thumb-sucking and masturbation will be discontinued as the child ceases to need the direct discharge of tension which they give him.

I have spoken here about children whose sensual development progresses easily; this happens when their bodily feelings are accompanied by fantasies which give pleasure without arousing too great anxiety. There are other children whose fantasies are associated with much fear and with feelings of guilt; their instinct tension is not so easily discharged and they are likely to suck their thumbs or to masturbate a good deal. As an example think of the hospital baby who during a period of overwhelming stimulation kept a precarious pleasure balance only by biting himself. At the time I was shocked by his biting because I knew that he would suffer for it afterwards, yet while he was distraught the additional pain in his thumb seemed to be the only thing that made his life endurable, and that is why I left him free to bite.

I want to make this point clear: that while sensuality always fulfils its prime use of relieving instinct tension and distributing feeling over different areas of the body, still it often happens that the means taken to relieve tension are opposed to the real interest of the individual. So it was in this case, for although the baby was calm so long as he bit himself he was finally left with a wounded thumb. Then he found his form of sensuality to be a two-edged sword. This is likely to be true wherever a child relieves great tension by exclusive stimulation of his own body. It is worth while to study the parallel cases of the child who sucks his thumb in season and out of season, and of the child who masturbates habitually, for so many parents are perplexed when they are confronted by the problem of strong instinct tension in their children. These are the very children who need to have things made easy for them and the parent has to decide what kind of policy will help them most.

Of course the persistent thumb-sucker is using mouth pleasure to relieve tension at a time when his contemporaries have more varied gratifications. Even so there is no reason to forbid it on the ground that he is too old to suck—not if he is four or eight years old, or any other age, for that matter. What we have to remember is that if the child sucks strongly enough to hurt himself or to make his teeth develop irregularly he is labouring under powerful general tension which forces him to go on sucking; if the mother forbids him to suck she may be actually taking away his most satisfactory bodily pleasure without finding him another one with which to ease his tension. As I see it an indication for limiting thumb-sucking arises when the child is actually in danger of altering the shape of his jaws, for then the parents will want to guard him against developing a rabbit face which would be a disadvantage to him in adult life. They will recognize, of course, that prohibition will inevitably raise tension and increase anxiety until the child has adapted himself to a new equilibrium; they must remember therefore to show him special favour and kindness while they interrupt the mouth pleasure that has satisfied him for so long.

This is a conservative policy with regard to thumb-sucking, and I think of the relief of tension by masturbation in the same kind of way. In most cases it is quite unnecessary to check it, for the child himself will deal with it appropriately. But if at the age of four or five he still masturbates frequently in the presence of the parents he is giving a signal of psychic distress and telling them

68

that some difficulty has arisen which prevents him from using his energy in ordinary play. A change of nurse or house often sets up transient trouble of this sort which is relieved as the child finds new interests, so that a kitten or a tortoise in the nursery helps some children through their difficult time and new supplies of plasticine or crayons help others.

Supposing that compulsive masturbation lasts over a long period, it is an indication that the child's fantasies are painful enough to cause him severe emotional strain; then the parents would be wise to seek skilled advice. They can also give support by being consistent in their attitude towards the habit, but there is no single attitude that is " right " for all children. It seems sensible to think of prolonged masturbation as a disability and to offer the child alternative pleasures ; if he accepts them, well and good. If, however, he cannot relinquish any of his genital stimulation it is unprofitable to nag about it, and a system of rewards and punishments will only add to his fear about the fantasies associated with it. Above all things the parents' friendliness to the child must not depend on his power to restrain himself from masturbating.

For a moment I want to return to the infant who finds his chief solace in thumb-sucking. Let us assume that things go easily with him ; he gets sufficient release from instinct tension, he is in no danger of pushing his teeth awry and the parents are quite willing for him to suck, so that no controversy and no feeling of guilt arises about his pleasure. Is it possible that indulgence in thumb-sucking can satisfy him and at the same time act adversely on his psychic development and adaptation to the world? I think it can, and in this way: if thumb and comforter are in use for hours on end they may jump the claim of other deserving household objects which are ready to engross the child. Then the thumb-sucking baby would learn little about boxes and buttons, ribbons and spoons, and though he might seem to be a comfortable and quiet child, still his tactile education would be woefully scamped.

At this point we comprehend a second use of sensuality; it urges on the baby to act and to make experiments on the world around him. For if he likes the look of a rattle dandled before him, he will want to suck it; if that proves satisfactory he must also grasp it, shake it, listen to it, bang it and suck it again. Every movement enjoyed leads him to make others, each one more adroit than the last. Then in the matter of sensation, from the very beginning each sense area has taken samples of whatever came within its reach; eyes were dazzled by light, fingers rested on a soft eiderdown, nose smelled the hot-water bottle as it dived into the cot. To begin with, the baby makes all these sensory experiments in a haphazard way. Let him watch as he waves his rattle and he will learn what it looks like; but if just then his eye is rolling elsewhere, the rattle leaves touch and sound impressions only—it has no colour for him and no shape, and can give him very little idea of the real thing.

By the fifth month, however, hand and mouth and eye are working together, and from that time onward this complicated sensory apparatus can be focused on every single thing that comes within reach to prove it and appreciate its quality. And with what result? Well, the child gains intimate knowledge of countless and widely different objects and at the same time a knowledge of the countless and widely different sensations he feels as he makes his investigations. He finds, shall we say, that a sponge has to be sucked if it is to be fully relished, while a newspaper must be crumpled and torn. And as he tears it he begins to understand something of its real nature, how although it is much bigger than he is, it can actually be crushed into a tiny space, and how it can hurt him only if he tries to swallow the bits.

These experiences of reality are based on sensation, and along with them there dawn in the mind fantasies, which are based on the same sensation. For the moment these crystallize round the newspaper and its properties, and, being stored in the memory, they become the very stuff of the child's psychic life.

Now while laying stress on the education value and the pleasure value of many and various sense impressions I have assumed that they are all agreeable and come from nice things. But what of the detestable sensations—those that come from too strait confinement in blankets, from soapy water in the eye and the open safety-pin? What use are they to the young child?

It is true that they enrich his range of sensation

and experience. They may also impinge on parts of his body that he hasn't yet recognized as belonging to him. Fingers may come to life in his consciousness by being entangled in a shawl and wriggling to get free—the foot, by being held too firmly when the mother washes it. By these sensations and reactions the baby learns about the parts of his body and the limits of his strength, just as he does about the things around him and their strength or weakness.

Another important use of painful sensation is that pain on the surface of the body can act as proxy for painful internal sensations or massive general sensations which are so much harder to influence or change. I remind you of the hospital baby who took grim satisfaction in the pain in his thumb and with its help somehow managed to bear his raging colic.

Painful sensations can be put to these various uses. I want for a moment to face one of their unfortunate results, and to see if it can be met in any way. The misfortune is that so few babies will experiment with a painful sensation, so they never find out what interests and charms lie behind it. I will give you an example of how good material was deplorably wasted because it gave one painful sensation to a two-year-old girl. I had painted some gay little houses, and gave them to her before the varnish had quite dried on the last one. " Sticky ! " she said with a curl of her lip, and never played with any of them again—and this although they were nice little houses giving infinite promise of good games. Evidently " sticky " meant to her something she must not touch, and this idea exaggerated her unpleasant feeling. But could anything have made the sticky sensation tolerable? Conceivably, if the houses had had chimneys and doors that opened she might have played with them. And in this way I put the case for a liberal sensual education; each object that passes through a child's hands has so many attributes that if it is loathed for one of them, in this case for stickiness, it may still be loved for others —for doors into which one can poke a finger or tall chimneys.

Parents can, in a sense, plan the liberal education of which I speak, for they can see to it that their baby has opportunity to cultivate unhindered his sense of touch and smell, sight and hearing and taste. And it seems to me that the child who has learned to use his sense-organs freely and with pleasure will be likely to take stock of the many attributes in his toys, and on this account to accept and play with them, although they may be sticky. And, as he accepts each one, he adds it to the armoury of things he uses to express his loves and hates and fears. Again the parents can help by resolutely accepting every toy and every attribute of the toy on the child's valuation. And in this frame of mind they should approach the mud-pies and puddles in the garden as well as all the things in the nursery cupboard. In the first instance, a smell is not a dirty smell but an exciting one, stickiness is not bad but interesting—and so it should remain as far as we are concerned. Every time we react with disgust or fear, the baby notices our disgust

and comes to suppose that stickiness is a bad thing
—exciting maybe, but bad, and to be avoided.   So
in course of time alongside the suspicious sticky sensation there will be ranged a multitude of allied
sensations which belong to the most desirable things,
and acting on our suggestion the " good " baby
may never allow himself to investigate them at all.
Thereby he will lose a lot.

An important practical question will occur to
you at this point.   Can we over-stimulate the baby
by offering him too many objects for investigation ?
I answer with certainty : he cannot have too many.
From the third month of life onwards he should
handle innumerable things.   But they should be at
hand in the cot or pram ready for him to pick up ;
they should never be forced on him, not dabbed
at his eyes and pushed into his tummie simply
because an adult wants him to take notice and play
nicely.   A forcing procedure such as I describe is
more like an attack on the child than a way of
educating him ; it is an instance of planned upbringing gone utterly astray.

Now when a young baby lies alone in his pram
playing with things, he usually begins by pulling
them to pieces, but as the weeks go on he learns also
to handle them with dexterity, and an early acquired
dexterity is of untold value to him.   This nimble-
fingered baby will soon make his toys do what
he wants ; he won't so often destroy them by mis-
chance—he won't therefore need to feel so guilty
about breakages ; finally, his parents will come to
lend him precious things like spectacles and watches,
so that he can learn what they, too, are really like,

74

and how he can use them for his practical and fantastic purposes.

Another practical point occurs to me. In buying toys for a child of three to four years the modern tendency is to avoid those which force him to play a certain game in a certain way.[1] He is left free to use most of his toys imaginatively and as he wishes. The same thing should hold true of a much younger child, and I think it worth while to make sure that every baby has at hand material which will introduce him to many sensations and will express many fantasies. He should handle big things among his little ones, hard toys among the soft, and things of the moment, like paper and flowers, among his solid bricks. He has a free range of toys then. He must also have free hand in playing with them. It is not part of our business to impose on him our way of playing cup and ball and our set of fantasies about that time-honoured toy. For our special baby the only right way of playing may be, contrary to general usage, to chew the string that joins the ball to the cup, and he should be at liberty to do it. There is no bad way of playing with toys. There are no sensations or fantasies specially to be sought or specially to be avoided.

Up to this moment I have spoken about tactile sense and experience, almost as if each object to be investigated could be applied to a passive baby, who then registered his sensations. A ridiculous notion, when in fact muscle activity gives exquisite

[1] Didactic toys certainly have their uses, but I would introduce very few of them into the nursery.

pleasure in itself and is the surest of all ways of discharging instinct tension.

As an example of muscle pleasure I remind you of the first essays in speaking made by a six- or eight-months-old child; how when he practises a fusillade of B's they intensify into spitting and popping which must make his lips tingle; how the E's go off into shrill peacock screams, and to the tune of those screams the vocal cords must strongly vibrate; how gutterals roll round his soft palate and the back of his throat.

By all these sensations the child discovers new parts of his vocal apparatus; as he co-ordinates their movements, he feels bodily pleasure—we hear as much—and in time he produces a voice that will get him what he wants in the world. In this way muscle pleasure, reinforced by the pleasure of listening, lays the foundation of the art of speech. And so, wherever one turns, it becomes abundantly clear that every sublimation, art or skill is built on a foundation of bodily pleasure, and specially on muscle pleasure.

Here again there is something to be said about the education of the senses. We cannot make a sluggish or ailing baby enjoy muscle pleasure by setting him on his legs before he is willing to walk. We have to recognize that one child has greater possibilities of pleasure in movement than another; but we can see to it that every baby is left as free as possible to use his limbs. For instance, there must be periods in the day when the infant wears no constricting napkin so that he can kick as much as he pleases; the toddler must race along on his own account when he wants to, and not always go walking hand-in-hand with his mother, and any impulsive movement, whether it is a movement of running or shuffling, snatching or banging, should be tolerated unless there is good reason to stop it. And this, because the child cannot develop full muscle pleasure from a movement which is frustrated. Put it in another way : the mother prevents her baby from rhythmically banging his rattle against the cot, and with that his pleasure is stopped. If it seems to him that she is forbidding him to make any kind of banging movement at all, and that she understands and condemns the fantasies which he was expressing with a bang, it is quite likely that he will neither recapture his " banging " muscle pleasure nor express his aggressive fantasies again in the way which was easiest for him.

I think you will have noticed a grave omission in this chapter up to now. When I said that the prime function of sensuality was to maintain a balance of pleasure for the baby, I did not mention the sexual feeling which is aroused by contact with people. Yet this is the feeling that can give more pleasure than any other. Again, in considering all the experiments in sensation that children carry out I ignored the fact that the things which excite them most are parts of people's bodies—the mother's breast and hands, the child's own bodily parts also, and especially the sensitive mouth, anus and genitals. Nor did I remind you that the smells of the body and its warmth, softness or hardness are far more stimulating than the smell of soap, the softness of silk or the hardness of wood. For not only do body smells, textures, and so on, stimulate the appropriate sense-organ in the baby, they also give him a general bodily pleasure, and when that pleasure is strong, sexual feeling is certainly associated with it.

I want now to discuss the sensual pleasure the child gets from bodily contact with people. Think of it as a general sensation; think of it also, at times, as intense local genital feeling. What is the use of these combined local and general feelings in the first six months of the child's life?

To begin with, we must recognize that during these early months the baby makes his most decisive reactions at his mother's breast, in her arms or on her knee—places which offer him much sensual stimulation. Some of the things he does there, like peaceful sucking, are delightful. Others distress him; such are the kicks and squirms with which he relieves his angry feelings and which quickly change into a kind of wrestling match with his mother. Other actions again, like excretory functioning, are emotionally toned as hateful or loving according to the child's mood. If he is angry, his motion will be designed to hurt the mother; if he is good-humoured it will be a gift to please her. But in every mood, angry or loving, his discharge of energy is associated with intense feeling which may indeed start locally but which immediately spreads over his whole body. I want to lay stress on the sudden and massive reactions of the young baby. The quick change in his facial colour and expression indicates how quick are the

changes in his mood; his sudden cries and movements suggest that whenever he is stimulated he is
bound to make an immediate and strong response.
As for the massive reactions, an infant often passes
his motion as part of a general muscle-contraction
which may be quite violent if the stool is hard; he
sometimes shudders as he urinates and when he
cries he struggles all over. When he is three
months old, his whole body is involved in every
action far more than it is a year later when appropriate groups of muscles are acting under his
conscious control.

It seems to me important that the place where
the young baby experiences his sudden and violent
changes in tension and feeling shall be a comfortable one, and, as I have reminded you, this place
is the mother's body or rather the embrace of her
arms. It must be comfortable in the sense of
offering new comforts and pleasures to the troubled
child, so that his rage and fear may be quickly
converted into emotions that are more tolerable;
comfortable in the sense of being placid even when
the baby is most angry; comfortable, finally,
because it is not too stimulating—for the baby has
plenty of his own tension to discharge without
having to deal with tension heightened by exciting
advances like tickling or dancing in the air. I
believe, then, that the earliest use of enjoyment
derived from the mother's body is that it makes a
medium which maintains a steady balance of
pleasure for the baby, and which does not accen-
tuate the extreme changes in his feeling.

Consider next the use of sensuality in the second

year of life. The bodies of the parents are not then regarded simply as safe or dangerous places in which the child moves ; they have become bodies of people with whom he is in love, and because he loves, he tries to imitate what he most admires in them. Thus a little girl lying alone in bed was practising the syllables " *oo-ell, oo-ell* ". She spoke them solicitously, and by this and the cadence of the sound I recognized the gentle " Well, well ", with which her mother used to comfort her.

A boy of two began suddenly to call his father " shavin' father ", so for him too the parent was a person who did special things. A week or two later the little fellow cut off his forelock with the nursery scissors, in this way imitating the shaving father, who happened to be also a bald father.

There is nothing strange in the lover thus taking the loved person as his ideal. The importance of this special result of falling in love in the second year of life is that while the child fashions himself on the admired pattern he begins to behave deliberately as a whole person—a very different behaviour from the impulsive reactions of infancy, when different parts of the body, mouth or arms or legs, acted independently because they were not yet fully co-ordinated. One could say that the whole personality of the child develops round his idea of what a parent should be.

There is a bodily change which is analogous to this integration of personality. It is the full muscular co-ordination which the child acquires about this time and which makes him able to do what he wants with his whole body. At last he can crawl along the floor to take possession of the people and things he likes, to escape from those he fears and to imitate the things that excite him. I remember setting a kitten on the floor at a little distance from a baby who couldn't yet crawl. She was terrified and could only lift up her arms for me to help her. A couple of months later baby and kitten met again. This time the baby imitated the kitten; she crawled round the room on all fours, and in body and mind she was that alarming little cat.

I always suppose that when this integration of body and mind has progressed some way the child is fairly well equipped to deal with big changes in the environment, such changes as the birth of a younger baby. It is easier for him now because his agility makes him independent so that he can get round the room to do and fetch what he wants on the spur of the moment, without having to wait for the mother to carry him about; his body serves him well. Moreover, if he has a clear picture in mind of how a kind parent behaves, there is a good chance that he will imitate the mother's care of the new baby and adopt it quite happily.

The love relation with the parents gives the child another kind of impetus to psychic development, for he tries so often to win their approval by new achievements and charms. He walks his first steps for their benefit, produces excretions to oblige them and tries to say words that they understand.

I feel strongly that the child should receive a due sensual response for all these things. He needs to be fondled and praised, and if the parents are unresponsive and lacking in interest they take away half the pleasure from his success. Sublimation still goes on, of course, without encouragement, but if it is not founded on a happy love relationship it is much more likely to break down in face of strain in adult life. And with that we come to one of the most difficult points in the planning of sensual education; for if the parents realize that they themselves are the richest of all the child's sources of sensual pleasure, they will give that pleasure freely, and the child will ask for it in the form of any bodily contact that is attuned to his fantasy—kissing, cuddling in bed and so on; this contact is his right.

But the parents' response must indeed be a response to the child's advance, and not a demand which is made because the parent is lonely and unsatisfied. To kiss and hug a child passionately cannot fail to excite him sexually, and it is quite impossible to know at what moment he is ready to deal with such excitement. Besides this, I believe that the parent who demands demonstrations of affection from the child may create in him a sense of obligation which should have no place either in the love that is natural in childhood or in adult life.

A further use of sensuality is illustrated by the behaviour of those children who make an insistent appeal for sensual satisfaction. When they are perhaps three or four years old, they are always climbing on the loved person's knee, kissing and asking to be kissed. But the children who need so much caressing are not gentle and clinging all the day. Indeed, the games they play during the time of heightened sensuality are generally more

violent than usual; besides, they behave tyran-
nously to other children in their group. A little
boy who was going through a stormy phase of this
kind met me for the first time and immediately
made shy and affectionate advances. At subsequent meetings he grew exacting and wanted to
climb up and hug me when I was reading or writing.
When he came to my room a few days later he said
he was a lion, so he roared and pretended to bite
and claw me. Soon he did bite me—I could have
avoided it only if I had kept him outside; when I
expostulated he said, " But I *love* to bite you "; said
it conclusively, as if it explained everything and
proved that both of us enjoyed the bite.

It doesn't need much skill to discover what use
these masterful expressions of love were to the boy.
When he hugged and kissed me he modified the
direct thrust of his hostility to me—nevertheless, he
contrived to stop my work. Forbid him the lion
games and what would have happened? The
aggressive impulse would not suddenly have faded
away, so it must have made its way out in open
rebellion against my authority and have brought
with it all the painful consequences of a bad personal relationship. But sensual pleasure did more
than help this child to discharge his tension in
rollicking games. It assured him that in spite of his
lion behaviour and the fantasy implicit in it that I
was a bad person fit only to be bitten, still I was in
fact a kindly creature with whom he could safely
exchange pleasant bodily contacts.

Here is the reassurance value of sensuality.
Every kiss, every caress the child gives proves to

him that he is good and pleases the parents. He needs no reassurance when he is happy and gives spontaneous kisses ; but the insistent sensual appeals I have spoken of bear witness to anxiety rather than spontaneity. They are desperate assertions that although the child would like to hurt the parents, still he can give them pleasure, if only by a bite ; and in this way he maintains a balance of love feelings over hate feelings. It is obvious therefore that parents should accept the various love advances with as good grace as possible, bearing in mind that the biting advance may be the only one that can be made for the time being. To fear the bite or any other manifestation of love or sensuality is to add very much to the child's own fear of his aggressive and sexual feelings.

I speak seriously of the parents' fearing the child's sensual demands, for it can lead them to adopt either of two unfortunate policies. Fearing any sensual advance they may strictly forbid it ; and if they do the child will not so easily make these advances in the future, even in the remote future of adult life ; or fearing sensual demands the parents may accede to them in all respects. If this should be the case the child may begin to plague those parents with his hugging or his curiosity, until he forces them to deal sharply with him, and the game ends in tears.

Now think for a moment of the provoking child. Actually he is more disturbed than exhilarated to know that father and mother are at his mercy, for him to treat as he pleases, and he is specially troubled if at the moment of his victory he feels little or no mercy towards them and actually has fantasies of biting them to bits. It may well be a comfort to him to know that they will not let him hurt them or love them too much; for if he is bound in this way to a certain moderation in conduct he need not expect sudden punishment from an exasperated parent, or from his own stern conscience. I therefore advise that in playing with their children the parents should stick to games that they themselves can share easily and with consistent good humour, for obviously their capacity for happy play will vary quite as much as the child's. Indeed, the parents' enjoyment of games should be one of the strongest environmental influences in the child's mental life.

So much for the pleasures and anxieties depending on contact with the parent. I want finally to look ahead and call attention to the influence of these pleasures on personal relations in adult life. I can make only a general statement about it; but I believe that if in his early love relations the child acts freely and meets with due response, he will go on expecting to love and be loved as the years pass —expecting also to trust people and to be trusted. And I think that once his body has found pleasure in contact with people, it will be prepared to find it there again. This is the happy sexual development we wish for our children.

IV. QUESTIONS AND ANSWERS

BY NINA SEARL

§1. INTRODUCTION

Some of the problems of upbringing, such as those given in the chapter on weaning, appear only at specific times ; some are dependent on the size of the family, for example, the problem of the only or of the youngest child ; others again are influenced by social or economic factors, the choice of a school is for the majority of parents limited by the length of their purse. But there is one problem which has to be dealt with by rich and poor alike, which appears and re-appears at all ages, which is often thrust upon us with a suddenness which may be disconcerting, and for which we cannot specifically prepare ourselves ; it is a problem common to parents, grandparents, uncles, aunts, nurses, teachers

and friends, which is therefore of interest to all—
the problem of a child's questions.

Not every question presents a problem. Many
are simple enough in themselves, and can be simply
and satisfactorily answered. Many, from their
freshness and originality, are a pleasure to the
questioned, and bring enlightenment to the
questioner. But undoubtedly a problem is often
recognizably present, whether it springs from the
number of the questions, their nature, the emotional
response engendered by them, the discontent with
which the answers are met, uncertainty as to how
far curiosity should be encouraged or discouraged,
or from any one of the many other causes which
may complicate the situation. Psycho-analytical
experience teaches us that a problem is often
present when parents and other adults do not
recognize it at all, and are content, for example, to
dismiss a child's question as " funny " or " queer "
or " just like him ". It is often there even when
an apparently simple question receives an apparently
adequate answer, and the child subsides.

We shall in the first place assume that the problem
is the child's and not the parents' (becoming the
parents' only from their desire to understand the
child's) ; it is important to know something of the
motivation of children's questions, and to make a
clear distinction between interest and curiosity.[1]

[1] These are not the only relevant distinctions, questions may
also spring from inquisitiveness and suspicion ; but if we can
clear our minds on the subject of interest and curiosity we are
well prepared for further discussion, and can regard inquisitiveness and suspicion as exacerbations of a central problem.

A person in a state of *interest* is in a quiet frame of mind. He is revolving in his thoughts the impressions he is receiving or has received from an object in the outside world, and in so far as it affords him pleasure, he finds this pleasure easily retained. Furthermore, he is not in a hurry and he is not specially impelled to touch or manipulate unnecessarily the object which excites his wonder. His interest tends to be sustained and is of a kind commonly called "receptive". In the state of *curiosity* we note that there is not the same quietness or peace of mind. There is an impatience to be doing something to the object, and an element of hesitation or doubt as well as of eagerness in the approach to it.[1] Interest is characterized by a relative freedom from fear, whereas in curiosity anxiety either impels or hinders. If the wish to obtain further knowledge were the sole motive for the child's questions, the problem would be an intellectual or an educational one in the narrower or "academic" meaning of the word, but experience shows us that this is by no means always the case; there are often emotional disturbances behind what appears at first sight to be an intellectual question, and nervous fears, doubts, and inhibitions complicate the picture, so that the problem is one upon which the psycho-analyst has something to say.

In curiosity, then, it is not merely a case of "I *want* to know about this", but also in varying degree "I *must* know about this, or I shall get into a panic"; there is always an element of urgency,

[1] Sometimes the hesitation and doubt are diminished and the urgency increased,

though this does not usually mount to such heights as to be pathological. We shall see later that it is this element of strain or urgency which gives all the trouble; it may arouse apprehension in the person questioned as well as cause disturbance in the child putting the interrogations, and so prevent his being satisfied.

§ 2. THE MOTIVES BEHIND QUESTIONS

A child's outlook is not the same as an adult's, it is both more realistic and more fantastic; realistic because he takes less for granted than do adults, departmentalizes his mental life less, and retains more closely the links with other more or less similar experiences—like an explorer advancing into quite unknown and possibly dangerous country, but retaining a connection with his base camps; fantastic because he is still often under the sway of emotions which can completely alter his relation to and understanding of his environment. Both his realistic and his fantastic outlook introduce difficulty in dealing with his questions, because they give them a content or significance for the child that is foreign to the adult. In addition, the presence of anxiety in his curiosity (an anxiety which proves him to be still struggling with past emotional experiences) prevents the child from gaining full satisfaction from even the most apt answers adapted to an immediate and to an intellectual experience. Lack of satisfaction increases the feeling of insecurity and the drive to investigation (if indeed the attempt does not succumb to discouragement and hopelessness), and either a predominantly fantastic, or an ultra-realistic outlook on the universe may be the permanent result. For if lack of a sense of security in the child's emotional relation with adults causes him to ask questions before he is old enough to appreciate the objective answer to them, he tends to link his new experience more closely with other emotionally similar experiences than with those whose similarities are of an intellectual order, the impetus of the question being emotional rather than intellectual. Here again, it is difficult to answer questions so that the child's intelligence shall not be overstrained in its endeavour to keep pace with, and thereby control this additional pressure of emotional experience.

I will illustrate from my clinical experience.

In the treatment room in which I see children I have an electric stove. During twelve years' repeated attempts to answer satisfactorily and to understand more fully children's queries about it, I have come to understand much that is hidden behind such questions, which in the ordinary way would not occur to the grown-up. Even if the latter did not understand much about electricity, he would have "placed" it in his mind in such a way that any remaining curiosity about its accepted familiarity would be concerned with what was peculiar to its individual working and different from other forces and objects—a comparatively unemotional situation. Little children, on the other hand, failing to grasp the simplest explanation about electricity, fall back mentally or emotionally on the question—the need to know—how safe they are with anything possessing such painfully dangerous possibilities. They become impatient and resentful at the unsatisfactoriness of a plain description, and endeavour to bring the stove and electricity into connection with other objects and situations similar in function, emotion and sensation. They want to know, for example, why the heat comes and goes so obediently and quietly, how it can be so easily and completely controlled by means of the simple movement of a switch, in striking contrast to a coal fire—and to so much else in their lives, including most frequently their own small selves. They wonder where the heat goes and where it comes from. The stove seems alive, at once dangerously hot and helpfully warm when alight, and safely but unhelpfully dead when out. They are not sure whom it is safe to trust with such a power of life and death, particularly a power of such assorted advantages and disadvantages, lest it be applied to persons as well as to stoves. In a deeper layer of their minds they sometimes think that the stove is a kind of silent reproach to them, telling them that they should feel hot with shame if they are as dangerous and inflict as much pain as can the stove, or if they are not as clean, helpful, quiet and obedient as it. They contrast it with a coal fire and do not understand how it can give heat and " burn " without consuming anything. They are not sure whether anything with such an evident avidity for burning and consuming if given the opportunity can be a safe companion when *not* given such an opportunity, and they feel rather than think, that it may be like a fierce unsatisfied animal or hungry child. Coal fires, on the other hand, consume dirty coal, and may seem to threaten dirty children ; but they only live at all fiercely when they are given enough to feed them, and quietly die down when left unprovided with food. The electric stove is clean, uniform and uneventful. The coal fire is dirty, but far more eventful and beautiful. In terms of that with which they are most familiar—themselves, and their own experience—this seems to tell them that the good clean child has a dull time in comparison with the dirty child. Possibilities of easy control and the pleasure in it restore some of the balance of advantage to the electric stove and the clean child. From the point of view of sensation, the hot " elements " are like that part of the body in which sensation is most vivid—the genitals. Reassurance conveyed by the fact that the " element " burns without being consumed fails them when the element cracks or fuses, and in any case seems only to apply to adults, since the stoves themselves never belong to children but only to adults. By their curiosity about and control of the stove they try to satisfy their curiosity about and desire to control these parts of adults' bodies, as well as to control the hidden and sometimes threatening emotions of both adult and child. In short, fuller understanding of the children's queries about the stove link it with the most significant and difficult of their previous experiences. And no amount of question and answer anent the stove and its working can satisfy that part of their minds which is considering it in quite other terms than that of " electric stove " alone, and is also trying to gain satisfaction and security from and control over something quite other than it, in terms of the stove.

Also in my treatment room I have a floor covered with green and white marbled rubber tiling. An adult considers it from an æsthetic or a practical point of view, if he gives it any special notice at all, and his æsthetic judgment is concerned with the general effect to which details are subservient, though they may be all-important from his practical standpoint. A child has not the same power of detachment in forming an æsthetic judgment. If he notices details and their variations from those of other floors, they may have an importance quite disproportionate to his general impressions; nor is the adults' practical outlook his in the same way. He does not as much want to know what are the advantages of such a floor in general or to the particular person, as what it can do for *him*, what it can tell him about a strange house, a strange room, and a strange person in that room; whether it will help or hinder his play, and so on. Often it is months before a child's first impressions are fully unravelled. If he had come into the room with a feeling of complete internal peace he would have been able to look at it with greater objectivity, even though his impressions would still not have slipped as easily into prepared departments of his mind as would the adult's. But children do *not* come into my room in a state of complete serenity of mind, and because of the tendency to projection whenever the mind is disturbed, the objects in my room become invested with much of the threatening significance of their own feelings, and the feelings, real or supposed, of other people. Therefore children want to know why the floor looks rather like a bathroom floor ; is it an indication of what I expect of them with regard to cleanliness ? or of what they may expect of me when they are there ? The manifest content of their question may be solely concerned with the flooring, but behind it lie thoughts about their personal relation to me.

We can follow the double-layering of the questions if we consider the way the children treat details. They wonder why the floor is cut into squares, for the more closely they connect the " bare " part of the floor with a bare body in a bathroom, and the more their own rages have made them want to attack people's bodies, the less they are able to think of the floor as *constructed out of* squares (real bodies, they know, are not made like that), and the more they feel impelled to think of it as *cut up into* squares, and they want to know what the divisions in the floor may indicate about their relation to me. They have a feeling of uneasiness that dirty people might not only be washed but be cut up in that room.[1]

If immediate circumstances and particular disturbances so add to the feeling of uneasiness that it becomes acute, the child wants to rush out of the room to something that seems less threatening, or he hurriedly turns to cutting up paper or other

[1] I mention these details to show that behind a simple question there are many problems which the child is trying to face, and that by his interrogation he is trying to find a solution to several at the same time.

material, or, if I fail to understand the early signs, tries to cut the rug. He must be active, not passive, for safety. If I am able to show him that I understand his fear of the cut squares, his uneasiness disappears, and the floor and I together once more seem harmless or helpful to him. If his anxiety is not too acute, he may, without words from me, use the lines forming the squares as something which furthers his play and pleasure instead of hindering it by apparent threat. Thus, playing in a way familiar to everyone, one child runs a toy car up and down the lines, another " puff-puffs " vigorously up and down them himself, and at another time, makes them a help to failing courage by playing at keeping ranks on them like a soldier. But it is characteristic of this anxious play that it is very liable to emotional interruption from within ; no interruption from without is tolerated, and the child easily becomes impatient and irritable. It is the psycho-analyst's work to know from the details of his present and previous play, from his talk and odd remarks, from his variations of attitude and expression, something more than either the general observer or the child is aware of. For example, from my previous knowledge of the boy who did the " puff-puffing ", I knew (1) that cutting and butchers' shops held a particular menace for him ; (2) that trains were mainly a menace, too, though also a help to getting where he wished (he hated and feared their noise and screaming whistles, and the impossibility of getting out of them when he wanted) ; (3) that he often used one danger to combat another.

Thus while the boy himself only knew that he felt very unsafe on that floor if he stopped playing at engines, I was able to tell him what other " pre-conscious " experiences he was pitting against one another, such as butchers' shops and noisy, forceful and imprisoning trains which could take him far away from the scene of danger, and why he felt he could only be safe if he himself were as powerful as an engine, keeping to the lines and not able to range anywhere and everywhere. From further details, such as one or two very angry and explosive expressions without context which were obviously copied from his father, I was also able to show him the more remote " unconscious " parts of his mind that were also expressed in his play—why he had come to regard his father as an embodiment of the most powerful and dangerous forces, and had understood engines in the same way, with the addition of remorseless lack of feeling ; why he felt safe with his mother and with me only while he was showing powers of secret control and direction over all threatening forces in himself and his father. When I interpreted these thoughts to him, his demeanour changed and the note of strain disappeared.

A child's play runs on three levels. The conscious one is in elastic contact with the environment; he uses objects that he finds about him for the purpose of representing elements in the situation he is imagining, such a situation being largely determined by the emotional needs of the moment. The second level, the pre-conscious, does not enter consciousness without some additional stimulus, such as my mention of butchers' shops and his experiences with trains. The third level is still more remote from consciousness. The significance of keeping to the rails, for instance, was completely unknown to the small boy while he was playing, as was the fact of his trying to control instead of reproducing his father's and mother's least amicable and most threatening relations to each other, and his to them.

The child's play springs from two sources ; one relates to the external and the other to the internal world. The same thing is true of children's questions, whose impulse, content, and emotional accompaniment may come from different situations and from different levels of the mind, but are always ultimately connected with the security of their relation to loved persons. Where they possess this security, children move trustingly through a world full of unknown dangers. Where they do not, they may feel unsafe in the most familiar and tried situations. Yet this relation, at its best, is liable to such sudden gusts of adverse feeling that the child's sense of insecurity is roused by any thoughts or feelings which, if put into action, might lead to the loss or injury of these loved people, or to the loss of their love and the capacity for loving them. Thus the child's security is liable to interruptions from within as well as from without ; and when he seems anxious without external cause we do well to remember this : he fears the power of his own thoughts and feelings. His naughtinesses and bravados do not contradict this fact, they confirm it. They spring from the difficulty of reestablishing safely and easily this lost or threatened relationship of love and security. So we must be prepared to find that the child has more need of reassurance than the adult, because he feels more beset by insecurity. Accordingly his questions will need to be met by an intuitive understanding of the levels of the mind from which they arise and the kind of anxiety they are designed to allay.[1]

To illustrate this point more fully I will return to the green and white marbled rubber tiling on the floor of my treatment room. Children generally approve of the green colour, but not of the white flecks on it. They may do no more than touch them with an investigating finger, they may ask no more—verbally—than " What are these ? " or " Why are they there ? " But from their attitude and facial expression, their tone of voice, their play and their other apparently quite irrelevant remarks, I discover how much more than simple inquiry lies behind these simple queries. Perhaps by some very careful arrangement of coloured bricks, with marked reluctance to their coming in contact with the floor, a child shows me that the flecks are, to her way of thinking, ill-arranged, and form no pattern, are merely untidy and without colour or design. My choice of them does not exalt me in her opinion. By her masterful request to me to pick up the fallen bricks from the floor, she shows me that she demands tidiness of me far more forcibly than I of her, and also demands that I

---

[1] Questions—those at least, which are not of an compulsive type—denote a certain freedom of the mind; absence of questioning may mark inhibition of thought.

should not allow her feelings to be upset or "untidied" by her dislike of my flecked floor. I tell her so and her play thereupon takes a much less reproachful and masterful turn. Another child looks doubtfully and suspiciously at the floor, and at me after a passing query about it, and perceptibly fingers a small spot on her hand, or glances at some spots on me. She, I find, thinks the white marbling is like a rash on a body, and particularly dislikes it because it reminds her of something seriously wrong, but she is too abashed at her thoughts to be able to put them into words. Another child flaps his arms and makes comical attempts to keep both feet lifted off the floor—he is trying to turn himself into a bird, and by his cursory references to the spots on the floor I know he is tactfully letting me know that to him they are like bird droppings, which he dislikes when he finds them on chairs in the park.

In all three cases, behind the apparently simple queries and these more elaborate and anxious references, lies a still more disturbing fantasy to which the cut squares have contributed—of a dirty or cruel person stronger than I or than my better self, who has mutilated and disfigured me and my room. If my answers to their "What is it?" had merely been "It is white marbling" or "They are just white marks on it," I should have answered the obvious or surface part of the question only, but not the far more important hidden content. To do this I had, as I have shown, to take into account the whole of the setting, not only that part of it which was immediate, but also what preceded and what followed the incident. And then, by way of other more or less loosely approximated situations, I came to understand that what they most urgently wanted to know was " Is there anything dangerous in the room ? ", " Are you a dangerous person ? ", " Is there any likelihood of my becoming dangerous to you or your room ? "

The full answer to these anxieties cannot be given without delving into the child's mind by a method that is not suitable for parents to employ on their own offspring—it requires a specialized and limited setting of its own, as well as a specialized technique. But the *attitude* to the question, the manner of meeting it can be shared by any and every well-wisher of children. If the remark about the marbling had been met by any implication of " How silly you are to ask such a question," if the acted or verbal connection of the marks with spots, rashes, or bird-lime had been met by the remark, " No, of course, it isn't that, don't be so nasty ! " the child would have felt an increase of anxiety and guilt, not only because of the consciously expressed thought, but because what was still hidden had been brought half-way to consciousness and then thrust back again in contempt.

We cannot be content with a classification of questions into those showing a scientific, a domestic, or an artistic interest. Such a classification may be satisfactory—and often subsequently extremely disappointing—to parents who are proud of gifted children, but it ignores the fact that questions are not the product only of an intellectual need for information, but are also a medium through which the child tries to adjust difficulties in his personal relationship. These two elements, the (conscious) intellectual, and the (often partly or wholly unconscious) emotional, are mixed in every case.

Nor shall we be satisfied with another type of classification to which parents and others are prone, which takes less account of the content and motive of the child's question than of its effect on the parents themselves; thus we hear of " exasperating ", " intriguing ", or " embarrassing " questions. These descriptions often reflect the parents' attitude to questions with more precision than the child's, but we must not be surprised to find that, possibly unconsciously, the child is trying sometimes to exasperate, intrigue or embarrass us. At its best the occasion may give him the opportunity of discovering that exasperation, intrigue and embarrassment do not create deadly enemies, and that it is possible to find another way of dealing with them than that he has hitherto discovered. But in any case, the key to the problem of this type of question is not in the intellectual, but in the social sphere, that of human relationships. A question is a social action in an intellectual form. When we think of an intellectual problem we turn our attention to its contents; when we think of a social problem we pay attention to its setting. With regard to questions, we should neglect neither their intellectual content nor their social setting; the *problem* does not lie only in the intellectual aspect of the child's question but also in the social relationships which lie behind them. With older children who have already achieved a fair measure of internal stability and independence, and whose anxieties are not a great burden to them, a question more often relates predominantly to the outer world, and can be satisfied by a direct answer. But with nervous children or with the very young, whose contacts with the external world are still uncertain and whose power of verbal expression is still very partial, the case is different. The emphasis is on the hidden content of the question, and they are only very incompletely satisfied if the question is met in a direct way. At this point let me emphasize that questions may come from more than one layer of the mind and usually do, that in answering the obvious part of the question adults should remember that another may be hidden beneath it, and that the child may be expressing his worry about his relations to other people and their attitude to him. Questions of either type should be answered with a friendly interest ; the more " queer " they are, the greater is the probability that a struggle is going on in the child's mind, and that our own mind is not seeing the problem in the child's setting.

§ 3. TO WHOM ARE QUESTIONS PUT ?

We have seen something of the variety of ways in which a child may make use of questions in order to restore his mental and emotional equilibrium. We have seen that this equilibrium is always, in the last resort, connected with the security of his relationship to some particular person. We need not, then, be surprised if the choice of person to whom the questions are put is determined not solely by propinquity, sympathy and intelligence.

(a) The little girl in my treatment room who expressed her reproach to me about the untidy marks, both non-verbally in her play with bricks, and verbally in her demands that I should pick up the fallen bricks for her and make the room tidy when she left—this little girl was at the time feeling worried about her bad thoughts and her rages of temper when I had occasionally thwarted her. Their invisible, intangible effect was still present in her relation to me, and because it was difficult for her either to disperse this unfortunate effect entirely or to grapple with it, she connected the uneasy feeling and the damage it was invisibly doing with visible details she did not like in my room. Therefore it was from me that she required information and reassurance about them. None the less, in her rages with me she had been re-enacting many other situations of thwarting she had both inflicted and suffered, and therefore there were other silent and invisible actors in her drama from whom she could not at the time gain the reassurance she wanted by question and answer. But the little girl was better able to put questions to them and to me for the sake of information and not for reassurance after she had proved with me the possibility of understanding the underlying anxiety.

(b) Questions can be put to other uses than the predominantly friendly one I have just described, even though the effort to maintain internal equilibrium by their means may be still there. They can be used, and with great effect, to extend a child's power over his elders. It is a fact familiar to us all that children often make obvious use of them to interrupt adult conversations when they cannot bear to feel excluded from them. I am thinking of the case of a boy who found that he could get his father's attention and keep it as long as he asked questions about trains or motor-cars or other mechanical contrivances in which his father was very interested, and he used the power thus gained to include himself in his father's interest and get it focused on himself to the exclusion of his mother. The motive for his questioning was a mixed one; it was not only to gain information. He exploited his father's own mechanical interests and his desire to have his son share them, in order to get more power over his father than his mother possessed, and to diminish the occasions of jealousy by keeping his parents apart. The more eagerness he put into his interrogations the more did his parents, who had no insight, think that they were promoting the mental development of their son. Years after, they may begin to wonder what had turned the boy away from an apparently early and marked proclivity for engineering, when all along his interest in mechanics as such was slight. A more impartial judge would not have based his opinion of the boy's aptitude on the number of his questions, but on their progressive insight into mechanical problems.

(c) In discussing the " exasperating ", " intriguing " and " embarrassing " questions we said that although these were classed according to the parental response, we must not be surprised to find that they often express the child's desire to exasperate, intrigue and embarrass. To this group belong those questions rattled off with great determination, rapidity, and force, fired at a target, as it were—the target being the person addressed. The choice of this person is determined by a feeling of resentment which would attack its object. None the less, although the accompanying hatred is clear in manner and expression, and although the compulsive element is conspicuous, the maintenance of the attack in the form of questions shows that the child does not believe that the door is definitely closed on him, and proves that he has not abandoned all hope. To remember this may be of some assistance in dealing with the particularly difficult situation, in which the motive underlying the compulsive questions is so largely unconscious.

(*d*) On subjects which excite a feeling of shame and guilt, and for questions which are inquisitive rather than curious, children will turn their attention to those who seem best adapted to keep their guilty and shamed feelings at a minimum. They will often seek information of other children, or of those in inferior social positions, such as servants, and not feel so free to go to those who may be best able as well as most willing to tell them what they want to know, but who on these subjects form the foci of their most poignant feelings. In such a situation it is a help to go to those who are less involved in the emotional situation, and who are not expected to feel ashamed of many things which may be conventionally anathema to drawing-room

standards. Social differentiations and varying codes
of behaviour often puzzle the child and excite in
him many queries he seldom sees fit to put. But
he tries to gain some advantage from them when
he is troubled by other puzzling queries which
would cause him shame and embarrassment if put
to those of more carefully regulated behaviour.

§ 4. RESPONSE TO QUESTIONS

The kind of response that questions evoke
depends upon the emotional state of the person
interrogated, and on his insight into mental processes. If, in his view, the mind is divided into
" reasonable " thoughts and actions and " unreasonable " ones, and if he views the latter with
contempt or uneasy irritability, he is compelled in
the interests of his own peace of mind to do all he
can to see and answer the intellectual problem, and
that only, in each question. And very heavily such
earnest, well-meaning and persistent endeavours
can press on the mind of the child, whose real need
utterly escapes such a person. The principal factor
in harmonious response is not knowledge upon the
topic in question, but the combination of an
emotional equilibrium with a kindly insight into the
mind of the child. It is hardly necessary for the
psycho-analyst to insist here on the importance of an
understanding of one's self. We cannot respond
freely and intuitively unless within ourselves we
have come to terms with the thoughts, feelings and
impulses which that question and the manner of
making it stir in our own unconscious minds.

Speaking generally, it is true of questions and

answers as well as of the more extensive problems
which Ella Sharpe mentioned in the first chapter,
that the pattern of one's behaviour towards a
younger generation is profoundly affected by the
pattern of one's behaviour in childhood towards
one's parents, and of their behaviour towards the
child of those years.

If a person in childhood used questions as a
means of attacking or separating his parents, he is
unlikely to respond easily or adequately when,
years later, much the same questions are put to
him by a child. He will still respond not to the
new and different situation, but to the earlier one,
which he has banished wholely or in part into the
unconscious. If his father replied roughly, he may
treat his own child in the same way, or on the
other hand he may be driven to make the situation
as different as possible from his own childish one
and answer every question as soothingly and suavely
as he can, blunting the points of the attacking
weapon, as it were. In such cases, whether the
technique be one of repetition or of reversal, the
adult is so apprehensive of the emotional factors
underlying the child's question that he is not free
to adapt himself to the needs of the child.

Turning to other types of response to questions,
I will illustrate what I have in mind by referring to
contrasting modes of behaviour.

(a) *Giving and Withholding*.

Some parents take a delight in answering a
child's questions, even to excess, often in striking
contrast to their grudging attitude about other

things, e.g. money, time for play, or food. They seem to have a compulsion to *give*, in the form of pouring out information, even to the point of fatiguing their small listener. We have seen how many unconscious motives drive the child to curiosity and how these factors complicate his internal life. If, in addition, he is also thus enticed towards curiosity, the resulting situation may well become unmanagable for him, however readily and eagerly he may seem to respond. On the other hand, there are people who grudge information, and dread to be asked too much, because they fear the child's easily aroused and violent emotions and his power to excite the same in themselves. They can seriously increase the anxieties of the child, who quickly senses fear of his own curiosity. He may either exploit his knowledge of that fear by tormenting the adult, or react to it with such guilt that the free exercise of his curiosity is prevented by internal factors ; that is, his curiosity is " inhibited ".

A very common difficulty occurs when children begin to read the newspapers and to push their questions beyond even the most sensational details given in the papers, inquiring minutely into details of startling accidents, and the injuries received in them, or into the exact setting of crimes of passion, or the motives of particularly sadistic assaults and murders. Sometimes they cannot let the topic drop, and later on perhaps have a bad nightmare. The parent does not want to damp down the child's curiosity, or to refuse information the child demands, and decision in such cases must always be a difficult matter. It must be adapted to the particular needs of the individual child; no general rule is possible; but it may be a help to remember that the anxiety prompting such insistent questioning cannot be allayed by repeated doses of the very type of information arousing it. The child is already making a rather despairing attempt to change that which he fears and hates into a pleasure. One should tell him enough to show that one is trying to further his own attempt to face his fears on the subject, and that when there is any good reason for knowing about such matters he need not be afraid to do so; but one can also convey to him that it is not necessary to know everything about them, or to take excessive interest in horrors and crime to show one is not afraid of them.

(b) *Solicitude and Indifference.*

Some parents are troubled by their children's questions, detecting the presence of anxiety, and, unable to respond to it wisely, they develop an attitude of great solicitude, fussing lest he is not answered well or fully, or lest he fails to question when he should. The effects of this on the child's mental health are comparable to those of over-solicitude about physical health. If the child finds his need of special attention sufficiently strong to overcome his dislike of its anxious and dominating quality, he loses spontaneity and independence; he comes to regard questions as a technique for placating anxious parents rather than as a route to understanding with the help of loving guidance what is going on in the world. The opposite tendency is for parents to treat their children's questions with blank indifference and neglect as if neither the questions nor the questioning child existed. Such parents may account for this behaviour satisfactorily to themselves, if not to the child, by saying that it helps the child to develop a healthy independence in solving his own problems. But any independence brought about in this way is likely to be of a revengeful and defiant type, which in its turn ignores the existence of the parents. Without keeping the child in a state of dependence on emotional, intellectual or moral problems, it is important to recognize that he needs help and has as much right to it as to food.

(c) Vexation at Questions.

Sometimes parents put on the armour of indifference as an alternative to a display of intense vexation and irritability at the searching questions of children. These parents would deplore as well as fear giving way to such an impulse as vexation, but are nevertheless unable to control themselves—and they do not know why.

For reasons concealed in their unconscious they are reacting to the children as if they were dangerous enemies, perhaps thieves and robbers trying to break into a closed house. But there is another unconscious defence employed by parents in which this situation is reversed. The children are not excluded, the parents do not resist encroachments on their privacy, but, more or less consciously, invite the child to penetrate every corner of their lives. They may think (consciously) that it is done entirely for the advantage of the child, but the fear of yielding to vexation plays a large part in such cases.

(*d*) *Respect for the Privacy of the Child's Thoughts.*

Sometimes parents think they detect, from their child's questions, a " complex " or other sign of " abnormality ", and immediately attempt to " explore the mind " of the child, thinking that their half-grasp of the elementary concepts of psychoanalysis will provide them with an easy means of removing from the child's mind what is disturbing to themselves. There are many reasons for appreciating psycho-analysis, but this is one of the worst. Or parents may seek to attain something akin to physical intimacy with the child through the most minute contact with his mind ; but if such an attempt succeeds at all it may result in an exclusive relationship which can give neither child nor adult what they unconsciously hope to derive from it. A child has a right to possess and a need to preserve the privacy of his own thoughts, and his emotional relationship to, and dependence on his parents should not be used by them as an opportunity to satisfy their own desires or eradicate what is disturbing to them. If a deepening of understanding is to be made the basis for a better relationship with the younger generation, the start, as Ella Sharpe has said, must begin within the self. If the child's questions reveal in himself and cause in his parents disturbance of mind, they had better apply to themselves any knowledge they possess of the unconscious mind, rather than begin to explore the unconscious mind of the child. We must show the same reserve in dealing with a child that we would show in dealing with an adult whom we love and respect.

§ 5. QUESTIONS ON SEX

In the last thirty years or so the attitude towards the sexuality of children has changed considerably. Before this they were regarded as having no interest in sex, or if they had it was thought to be either abnormal and something to put a stop to, or else a premature intellectual interest that could be best dealt with after they grew up. But lately, partly owing to the influence of Freud, sexual questions have come to be regarded as a normal expression of a child's curiosity, a child's sexual activities are looked upon with less horror, and as a consequence, children can more openly ask questions on such subjects. Previously, with the object of sparing children the dangers of sexual knowledge, every mention of its existence was suppressed; now it seems to be thought that a child cannot be informed young enough or thoroughly enough on "the facts of life". It seems, indeed, that the earlier solicitude lest the child should show premature curiosity on the subject has been converted into solicitude lest he should not show it early or fully enough.

There is a well-known story of the little girl who was heard murmuring to herself after an informative talk from her mother, "Yes, it's quite true as Mummy says that babies grow in the mother's tummy, but it is *also* true that they are found under gooseberry bushes." Something had gone wrong with her sexual education; it is fairly clear that " the facts " were not being assimilated. The explanation for this state of affairs lies in the fact that the child was prevented by her own conflicts from accepting the truth as she knew it and as it was told her, and from rejecting and condemning as a lie the untruth which had been told her.[1] In addition the gooseberry bush story serves a useful function in the child's mind. The displacement of the site of gestation serves to reduce the tension *vis-à-vis* her mother in another way also, for the vegetable theory puts aside the objectionable notion that the baby has resulted from a physical intimacy between her parents. A child's lack of comprehension of what are called " the facts of life " is frequently due to hindrances originating in jealousy, hatred and the feeling of loneliness and insecurity.

Should the child's questions about sex be answered? (Whether we know it or not, whether we like it or not, they will be taken as answered in some degree whether we treat them with silence or with lengthy explanations, with avoidances, or with eagerness. That is, the child will in any case become aware of our emotional attitude to them.)

Before we answer this with an unconditional affirmative we should consider more closely the nature of the situation in which his questions are

[1] A child's tendency to be gullible and credulous is often the result of a need to preserve other children and grown-ups from the rigorous and aggressive judgments of early childhood on those who do not speak the truth.

put. Is the child totally ignorant of sexuality, and does his question indicate a void to be filled up ? Or has he some knowledge and is he puzzled by certain aspects of the matter and therefore needs to get it straightened out in his mind ? Or is he worried about some of his own sexual and emotional feelings and thoughts connected directly and indirectly with sexuality, so that he wants to be reassured that these sexual feelings are not dangerous or wicked in himself or in his parents ?

Now how are we to know which kind of question it is that is being put ? I offer the following tentative suggestions. If the subject of the question fits into an obvious and natural context and the question is well put, the child is getting *facts* straightened out. For instance, if on seeing a cow and calf in a farmyard a child says, "Does the calf come out of the cow in the same way as the kitten comes out of the cat and a baby out of its Mummy ? " the probability is that the child is ordering or classifying sexual phenomena without much anxiety, though this is not certain. In general, a question expecting the answer " Yes " indicates less hidden anxiety than a question expecting the answer " No " ; but if, soon after receiving an affirmative answer, the child asks the same question again, it is clear that something is bothering him. We must therefore modify the foregoing generalization by adding that when a question is repeated soon after it has been answered, whether the answer expected be " Yes " or " No ", it is an indication of anxiety, and if the " No " answer is needed as a reassurance the worry is probably greater than if a " Yes " answer is repeatedly needed.

We get some light on the psychological situation if the child looks worried when he asks the questions. We must read the expression on the child's face and take that into account as well as the verbal significance of his questions. We sometimes hear parents complain that their child harasses them with interrogations, without a word about the child's own harassed looks at the time.

Another way we can get knowledge of what is behind the question is by noting the moment when it is put. Sometimes a child will let his parents' idle moments go by, but will begin his questions as soon as work begins. (If he chooses that time to ask when the doctor is coming to bring him a brother or sister, we may fairly safely infer that he is reluctant to have that anticipation realized.) So long as he is free to have his parents' uninterrupted attention he can stave off his jealousy, and even banish the worries from his mind ; but as soon as he feels that he has not undisturbed access to his parents' attention he must do something to demand it in order to avert the return of his mental strain. Only in the rarest case will a child be satisfied with one question in circumstances such as these. He will put a second in order to see that the quiet, matter-of-fact attitude of his father has not been ruffled by the first interrogation ; and a third and a fourth, not so much for the sake of an answer in words, as to extract from the tone of voice in which the answer is given the reassurance of which he stands in need, that is, that he has not brought about his own exclusion from his father's mind, instead of that of the rival (for the moment the work) which he has been trying to exclude by his questions.

The fact that the child continues to assert the gooseberry-bush theory after being told of the uterine origin of babies should not lead us to a cynical or discouraged attitude to answering his questions. It is a valuable support to his own observations to have his *correct* sexual theories confirmed. We must recollect that the child's intelligence is not so very different from that of a scientist exploring new fields and devising new theories ; he has many hypotheses to account for the observed facts and is kept busy selecting the best ; it is difficult for him to be objective and it is always a comfort to have another observer who will share the labour of making observations and help with an opinion. The parents are obviously vested with great authority on this subject and should answer the points put by the child, that is, should on request state the facts. But should they do more than that ?[1] Much has been said about anxiety and insecurity. Should they take steps directly to remove these disturbing factors ? Let us look at the difficulties in so doing.

When the work of investigation and inquiry is being carried out predominantly by the less developed parts of the child's mind, he cannot act toward his hypotheses as does the true scientist. If anxiety is in

---

[1] We are excluding from the scope of this inquiry the approach of puberty, when, still paying kindly regard to their children's reticences, parents should make sure that boys and girls are familiar with the main outlines of sexual knowledge.

the ascendant, he does not choose the best, that is, the most in accordance with the facts, but rather the one that appears the safest for his precarious and oscillating emotional balance. It is quite obviously useless and unwise to combat with intellectual vigour erroneous views which thus seem to the child essential for his safety. Our only means of deciding whether we are likely to give more help than hindrance is the incidence of the child's own request for information and the setting in which it has been made, which leaves us much where we were before. We should give the child the support for his observations for which he asks, and no more than that (although we should never respond to tentative inquiries with the impression that on our side the subject is closed when the answer has been given).

Parents need much wisdom in tackling disturbing factors if they are not to run the risk of leaving the child's equilibrium in a worse state than it was before. Once the disturbing factors form any organized part of the mental life, parents can do little about them in any direct fashion, though fortunately they are still able to do a good deal indirectly. If we remember that the crux of the matter is emotional equilibrium, we can see where they can give the most certain help, for sex problems will become less disturbing to the child if they show him by their own attitude that, without either ignoring or hiding sexuality, it is possible to maintain their own mental poise. The child's problem of emotional equilibrium is ultimately one of the security of his love relations, and as, in the effort to retain these, he often becomes a very tense and ardent little lover, they should not parade before him unnecessarily the facts and the pleasures of sexual relations from which he is excluded. But neither should they go to the other extreme and hide or ignore the pleasure factors by giving him the sexual facts for which he asks only in the guise of biology, for instance. We do not really deceive him by so doing, for, in so far as his mind is open to the truth at all, he has his own sensations and emotions to give the lie to such an attempt, and we therefore only shake his belief in our sincerity. After all, the mainstay of a secure relation between children and ourselves is honesty, which until recent years has been allowed small scope in dealing with their sexual problems. In these days we perhaps need to remind ourselves how even a few years ago deceptive theories such as that of the gooseberry bush were almost universally considered correct fare for children's hungry minds. Furthermore, we should not give him the impression that knowledge of the facts of sex gives to grown-ups complete understanding of the mystery of the creation of life ; such pretensions entice his intellectual powers to attempt more than they can possibly accomplish, at a time when the demands of the unconscious are impelling them in the same direction. The result can only be a sense of inferiority and discouragement.

Avoidance of the whole subject of sex leaves children with apparent confirmation of their hidden fears and fantasies, with the sense that sexual matters must really form a body of dangerous mystery which cannot be approached without great risk. This feeling of risk often shows in unexpected ways, and is sometimes hidden behind a bold front. A little girl of six once asked her analyst quite wistfully and in all seriousness, with obvious envy in her tone, "Do *you* know what it is to be a ' bashful maiden '? " This child had displayed the most unabashed curiosity on sexual matters, and had received all the information she asked for. She had not merely *wanted* to know, but had felt she *must* know, to prevent panics. And in order to remove some of the difficulties of dealing with a subject round which her anxious fears gathered it had seemed necessary to act as if she were completely intrepid. Shyness and bashfulness were too great hindrances and made her too vulnerable. She did not want to feel bashful—a feeling she dreaded —but she did want to be *capable* of feeling bashful, instead of being dominated by her apprehension of danger.

So much, then, about what we can do and what we should not do to help children struggling with factors which disturb their powers of observation. But in planning for the future, still another way is open to us. We can do something, if not every-thing, to prevent the *inception* of such factors in the mind of the child. I will not go into general matters which do not affect the subject under discussion more than they do every other depart-ment of the child's life—love, wisdom, patience, understanding, and so on ; but will single out two factors particularly germane to it—over-stimulation on the one hand, and deprivation of early sensual experience on the other. This subject has been dealt with in the previous chapter. Here I will only say that a certain amount of loving physical contact, besides that given by breast-feeding, is quite obviously the child's right, and that he may later try to compensate for an early lack of it by excessive demands for it, unless indeed he becomes inhibited. In either case we have results very similar to the outcome of over-stimulation, which are, in general, either inhibition or premature demand. The child's response to either insufficient or excessive physical stimulus being to make active demands for compensatory or excessive and premature physical satisfactions, his undeveloped powers of intelligence and control are over-taxed in the endeavour to maintain the psychical equilibrium of the total personality. His way of overcoming past difficulties may be either by compulsive curiosity or else by its inhibition.

It is more important to plan how to bring up children with the minimal number and intensity of disturbances than to plan how to deal with these when they are in being, and some grasp of the reasons which underlie the suggested ways of preventing and dealing with them is far more important than advice about specific instances in itself. We want such a comprehension of the factors involved that we are ready to apply our knowledge to the immense variety of occasion for which we shall certainly need it. And it is, I trust, unmistakably clear that we want more than knowledge for the purpose. The most accurate knowledge will be useless unless it can be applied with a kindly understanding which is free from unconscious complications, distortions and " blind spots ". This is the all-important factor in the situation. In this chapter we have talked much about anxiety, and insecurity, about disturbing and obscuring factors ; scarcely at all about situations in which these are absent and in which children and adults have a happy freedom of question and answer. The fact of this omission illustrates the belief implicit in psycho-analytical practice, that we only need to deal with the impairment of function, with that which impedes, deflects and exaggerates it, and to prevent and remove such impediments, for it to be spontaneous and accurate.

V. HABIT

WITH PARTICULAR REFERENCE TO TRAINING IN CLEANLINESS

BY SUSAN ISAACS, C.B.E., M.A., D.SC.

THE subject of habit is a large one. Not only do particular habits play a large part in the life of most human beings, but there is in many people a strong tendency to cling to habit as such, for themselves and for their children, as a bulwark against unwanted ways of behaviour. It is of course a common experience that a well-established habit is very hard to change, whether it be good or bad. We feel secure, therefore, if we have built up a series of useful habits for daily life in ourselves, or " implanted " them in our children.

Many people seem to feel that the key to the whole education of little children lies in inculcating good habits and avoiding bad ones. Some of the clinics in America which deal with the difficulties of little children actually call themselves " Habit Clinics ". Most books for parents and nurses include a chapter on " Habit " or on " The value of good habits ", and the chapter headings of one well-known book on the training of children speak not merely of " Habits of Eating ", " Habits of

Sleeping ", and " Habits of Elimination ", but even of " Habits of Play ". Some educationists regard even the major virtues, such as truth-telling, to be mainly a matter of habit, which if once built up will guard one against untruth in circumstances of stress and temptation.

Perhaps it is in the modern practice of infant welfare, however, that we see the doctrine of habit most plainly illustrated. Practically all the text-books dealing with the psychological care of infants and very young children lay the major stress upon the necessity for regular routine in the infant's life and the setting up of regular habits with regard to feeding, sleeping and excretion. It is said that " one cannot begin too early " to train regular habits in these directions. Such a view was expressed long ago by Carlyle, when he spoke of habit as the " deepest law of human nature ", and " our supreme strength. . . . Habit and Imitation are the source of all Working and Apprenticeship, of all Practice and Learning in this world."

Not only have practical people and some philosophers been inclined to give habit such a value. In recent years certain experimental psychologists have also inclined to this view. The American behaviourists teach that the education of the child is entirely a matter of " conditioning " his reflexes, that is to say, of setting up specific habits of this or that sort. They claim that there is no limit to the power of such acquired habits ; and that there is indeed nothing in the mind of the child or adult but these. This extreme view is held, however, by only a small number of experimental students of the child's development. The great majority even of those who agree that habit is important would also hold that it is but a mode of expression of certain fundamental drives or instincts which lie below its surface. The behaviouristic view of human nature is open to many serious scientific criticisms. Into these, however, I have no time to go, and will content myself with saying that such a view arises largely through faulty methods of observation and experiment.

It is not to be denied that habit is of practical importance. The problem before us is that of understanding what habits mean to the child himself. It is the special privilege of the psychoanalyst to see these things from the inside, to discover the feelings and wishes and fears and fantasies which are crystallized into a particular habit. And it is this aspect of the mental life, the unconscious psychical significance of habits, which concerns us in this chapter.

The problem has two major aspects. First, that of the regularity of the infant's life as arranged by the parent, in other words, the habits of the parent and the meaning of these habits to the child. You will remember that this aspect of the problem was touched upon by Miss Sharpe in Chapter I, when she spoke of the implicit plan of life of the parents and the way in which this might affect the child. I shall return to it myself in the next chapter when we discuss " The Nursery as a Community ". The other chief aspect is that of the child's own habits, whether they be the " good " habits we encourage, or the bad ones we deprecate and try to get rid of.

It is therefore *the habits of the child* with which I shall mainly deal now.

The previous contributions to this symposium must have helped to make clear to you how much more there is in even the young infant's mind than mere reflex response. Mrs. Klein mentions of some of the profound psychological meanings of the child's suckling, of his impulses towards his mother and her breast, and of the special significance of the process of weaning, with all its rich feelings and fantasies. Dr. Middlemore speaks of the comfort which the child so often finds in habits connected with a particular part of his own body, for example, in thumb-sucking or masturbation. She suggested to you that this bodily pleasure helps the child, both by building up his belief in the possibility of real satisfactions, and his trust in the goodness of his mother, and by reassuring him against his fears of loss, his anxiety about his own wishes to bite and scratch, and his unconscious fantasies of punishment in like kind from his parents. You are, however, already aware how far from the truth must be any notion that such habits are an affair of simple reflexes, and what a wealth of significant psychical experience may be summed up for the child in this or that apparently simple bodily habit.

Moreover, it is not only true that a particular habit is for the child a defence against a particular unconscious fantasy or wish. His clinging to habit as a whole may be one of his main defences against the anxiety connected with aggressive impulses and fantasies in general. You know how many infants resist any change of routine, whether it be a different time of day for a meal or a sleep, a different order of dressing and undressing and bathing, or a different person or place. With some infants and small children this is very marked. They seem to feel insecure and terrified if the accustomed routine is changed in any particular. Such an attitude is the counterpart in the infant himself of our own, when we cling to habit as an ideal for him, and it has the same roots. The child feels that any change is likely to be a change for the worse; at the least it stirs up a feeling of grave uncertainty, which is in itself very unpleasant. The foundations of the world shake, and it may fall. Parents cannot be trusted if they do not behave in the same way from day to day and moment to moment. One cannot trust oneself unless things are constant. A habit of order and cleanliness in given circumstances can be adhered to, but if the circumstances are changed, the door is opened to uncontrollable impulse and immeasurable dangers.

This protective function of habit in general will occupy us again in the next chapter. For the present, it will probably be most useful if I take one of the particular fields in which habit is specially emphasized as a valuable thing in training. It is with regard to problems of feeding and weaning, of cleanliness and of sleep, that good habits are so much stressed. The problem of training in cleanliness, in particular, occupies a large part of the time and interest of mother and nurse and child during the first four years. It is a question about which mothers and nurses are often very troubled, and I have gained much of my own appreciation of the child's difficulties in this connection through discussing them with mothers and nurses. There is no aspect of nursery life which is more intimately connected with the happiness and unhappiness of the family. The problem of training in cleanliness may be considered under three main headings :

I. The mother's aim, and the generally accepted views as to how this should be achieved.

II. The problem as seen from the child's side, and his difficulties.

III. The suggestions as to methods of training which psycho-analysis has to offer.

I. It is natural enough that the mother should wish to ensure the efficient action of bladder and bowel in the child for the sake of his bodily health. But for her own practical convenience she wishes also to ensure this action at a given time and place. Now it is obviously very much easier for the mother or nurse if the child can perform his excretions in an appropriate place and at a specified time. This real ground for wanting the child to be trained is not to be gainsaid. There is, however, a more potent reason than this for the great emphasis so commonly placed upon early cleanliness. The mother is not merely inconvenienced ; she is ashamed and anxious and morally indignant if the child is not clean at a certain age. She regards it as a social reflection upon herself and may even fear he never will become clean and orderly if he is not so by a given age. But these strong feelings of fear and shame and indignation are by no means so justified as might appear at first sight. They arise to a greater extent from the mother's own unconscious fantasies than they do from the objective facts of the child's development.

It is natural enough that a mother should feel ashamed of a child beyond a certain age who cannot control his bladder and bowels, just as she would feel ashamed if she herself could not. But it is obviously important to know what that " age " is, when children can be expected to be clean and controlled. In recent years, we seem to have been shifting the age when we make this demand further and further back towards early infancy. Many inquiries come to me from mothers who are extremely agitated because a child of fourteen months, even ten or eleven months, is not yet clean and dry. It is obviously very important to have a proper standard in this matter, a standard based upon real possibilities.

With regard to methods of training, the most common view nowadays is that there should be regular habituation to a vessel at specific times from the very earliest days. It is asserted that such early and regular training of bladder and bowel leads to a settled habit of cleanliness which will remain secure all through the later years. I may quote from a well-known book on the care of the baby.

> The first of these good habits should be initiated soon after birth. Twice daily after the morning and evening bath the stimulus of the cold rim of a soap dish or other little vessel should be applied to the buttocks, the abdomen should be gently rubbed at

the same time. . . . This stimulus must be *absolutely* regular and will soon provoke the required response, and will then be a good habit which has far-reaching effects. It will last through childhood (although fixed times for the child to "sit down" must be strictly adhered to), and into adult life, and is *one of the best preventives of constipation.* . . .

Most children can be taught to dislike a wet napkin, and by 7 or 8 months old can often discard it in the house, only wearing knitted drawers.[1]

It is quite generally taught in the text-books of infant training that this attempt to establish early habits is successful, apart from exceptional cases. Mothers have generally accepted this teaching in the most docile way, and go to endless trouble to carry it out, persisting in effort both for themselves and for the child whenever they do not have immediate success. They feel that it shows some abnormality in the child, or some failing in themselves, if things do not turn out according to plan, and they try this and that way to enforce the habit, always trying to get the child to function here and now, so that the habit may be established. The child may be kept on the pot in an uncomfortable position for twenty minutes or half an hour at a time, or scolded or reproached or smacked or bullied, anything to get him to conform to the ruling of the text-book which says what he should do and when he should do it. And if, after all this, things do not go according to rule, both mother and child become exasperated and despairing.

[1] Hewer, *Our Baby*, p. 97.

It is clear that this practice treats the child's
sphincters as local mechanisms which can be stimulated to reflex action irrespective of his feelings
and attitudes as a whole. Holding him over the
pot or sitting him on it, glycerine suppositories,
enemas, etc., are supposed to be the appropriate
stimulus to this local reflex action. Some even
advise a suppository for actual training.

> A soap-stick or glycerine suppository may be used in
> beginning training in order to condition the child.
> The use of a suppository should be clearly distinguished
> from the use of enemas or laxatives, which should only
> be resorted to on a doctor's orders. The suppository
> is merely a mechanical means to stimulate the sensations
> and movements appropriate to the act of defæcation.
> Its use helps the child to recognize incipient pressure
> and to facilitate the movement by voluntary effort.
> Suppositories should not be used for more than two
> weeks at a time. A child may show violent resistance
> to their use. If the case is one which has presented
> persistent difficulties, the resistance must be dis-
> regarded—it is almost sure to disappear with repeti-
> tion of the process. On the other hand, if, in the
> initial stages of training, strong resistance develops, it
> may be better to train the child by watching for the usual
> time for movements to occur and then anticipating by
> putting the child on the chair just before that time.[1]

It almost seems to be implied in this practice of
inserting a soap-stick as a means of " training ",
that there is no natural connection between the
sensations and movements in the colon and the

[1] W. E. Blatz and H. Bott, *The Management of Young
Children*, 1931, pp. 133-4.

sensations and movements in the rectum. In other words, that the physical intervention of a foreign body is necessary to make this link for the child, and bring the process under conscious control. This is surely a quite unwarranted view; it is both biological and psychological nonsense. And the practice is both unnecessary and undesirable. Fortunately, this particular view as to the training of the sphincter is not widely held, although many people do teach that a suppository is a useful aid for combating habits of constipation—a point which I shall discuss later.

The essential theory underlying all this emphasis on regular stimulus and regular opportunity from the earliest possible age is thus that the action of the bladder and bowel is a local reflex mechanism which can be " conditioned " to a particular stimulus, independently of the child as a whole or the situation as a whole, or of the age of the child. The effect of the child's emotional attitude to his mother on his muscular control of bladder and bowels is entirely overlooked or denied by those who speak in this way of " conditioning " or training. They fail to recognize that in the controlling or giving out the child is expressing a mental function by the medium of his sphincters. The text-books speak of what they consider the child's response ought to be according to the theory of reflexes, and notions derived from this theory about regular and easy " good habits ". We have, however, only to observe the actual experience of mothers and nurses to find ample proof that the practice breaks down and that the underlying theory is false.

II.   Let us now turn to the child's point of view as it is shown to us in the descriptive facts of his behaviour, and in his unconscious fantasies as revealed during the work of analysis.

During many years' experience in helping mothers and nurses about this problem I have gathered a wealth of descriptive material of the struggles of the child in his effort to gain control of his bladder and bowel during the first five or six years of life. A number of infants, not very many, fail altogether to respond to the early training with a vessel. Far more commonly the infant does respond to the early training in a way that seems to bear out what the text-books say and that proves to be most convenient to mother and nurse. He appears to be perfectly trained and clean up to, say, ten or twelve or fourteen months of age. Then comes a change, not by any means in every case, but so frequently that I am beginning to think it is a typical happening. The child begins to be dirty once again. Either he refuses to use the pot altogether, or he will use it for bladder and not for the bowel, or the reverse. Here are some examples quoted from the actual letters or descriptions written to me by mothers and nurses about particular children in good middle-class homes :

> She (aged 16 months) was trained from birth to be a clean baby, but within the last two months she has persistently fought and screamed every time the chamber is produced. When she comes in from the garden she is immediately held out, but I can never get her to do anything—and she does nothing but pinch me and go perfectly stiff on my lap. Then after

she has played around for a few minutes she will wet herself, and looks up at me as if she knows that she has been naughty.

From 4 to 10½ months I never had a soiled napkin, then at that age we took him on holiday. From the first day he changed completely—refused to use a chamber, but stiffened and screamed every time he was held out. He waited till I had put a napkin on, then wet or soiled it, and has done so now for four and a half months, though I have always held him out as a matter of routine.

Every night my son (aged 3) wets the bed, and wets his trousers during the day and frequently makes a mess in them also. This dirtiness during the day is quite a new thing, as he had been clean for many months now.

My baby boy, aged 2, has suddenly, after having been practically perfectly clean in his habits since he was a year old, taken to wetting his trousers. Smacking has not helped—in fact he comes up to me and in my face, though with no defiance, he says, " Mamma, I'm wee-weeing." When I say angrily, " What will Mamma do now ? " he says, " Give me a good smacking." He gets it, but an hour later repeats the performance.

When she (3¼) started teething she began waking up during the night every two or two and a half hours. Then several months ago, having been perfectly clean in her bed for a year or more, she began wetting the bed, sometimes once, or as much as two or three times every night, without any apparent reason—and as yet shows no signs of stopping.

My little girl, aged 13 months, is very tiresome about using her pot. She has always been held out before and after meals ever since she was born; and for months, in fact until a few weeks ago, we never had a dirty nappy (as distinct from wet). Now she is always wet and dirty as well. I used to hold her on my lap, but she fought to get off, so now I sit her on the floor on it, but she just sits there and does nothing, and after she has had her napkin on for about ten minutes she does it. She is bright and intelligent for her age, very well and happy. I haven't smacked her or done anything about it except try and catch her when she wants to do it. Is it best to just leave it and go on trying or ought I to scold her? Surely at her age she ought to be clean.

Perhaps these few instances of children from different families are enough. I could multiply them many times, but I am sure that nearly all mothers could supply examples from their own children.

One naturally wants to know what causes this breakdown in the sphincter control which has once been achieved. The answer varies. Sometimes no external reason can be traced. In other cases, it is clear that a particular happening has stirred up the difficulty, for example, a change of general routine, a change from the bottle to solid food, a change in the time of the midday rest, going away for a holiday, teething, the birth of another baby, the mother's illness or miscarriage, the loss of a nurse and coming of a new one, and other such significant events.

The child nearly always responds to such situations with strong feelings, but the mode of response is an individual matter. Some show grief and terror, some become suddenly obstinate. Others become generally anxious, and in many the fear takes on a specific character, having particular reference to the use of the pot. I may quote some further letters illustrating the stress of anxiety which the child may feel about this.

My small son (15 months) has taken a dislike to his pot and I think that it is probably uncomfortable for him. He seems to feel unsafe and clutches my hand when he is seated, also yells loudly. I have never pressed the use of a chamber and this is the first little bother I have had with him.

The trouble is that she (3½ years) persists in waking all through the evening and night wanting to use her chamber. I recently had a fortnight's holiday and unfortunately Jean was not lifted at 10 p.m. one night, resulting in a wet bed the next morning. She was very ashamed of herself and is so frightened that it will occur again. All our methods to cure this seem of no avail. At first we tried letting her have her chamber all through the night whenever she wanted it, but this seemed to have no effect and she was missing such an amount of sleep. Then we tried to make her wait for definite periods, e.g. if she cried during the evening we said she must wait until nanny came to bed, etc., as was usual. She would ask for it about two minutes after she had used it. If we did not give her the chamber she would scream and get really worked up. One evening she screamed for two and a quarter hours. We now put her chamber beside her bed and tell her to get out and use it when she needs it. The result of this is that she is continually out of bed, all during the evening and night. Like this she is missing the best part of her night's rest, and of course she keeps me awake every night too. . . .

I might add that she is having a baby sister or brother next month. She has known about it for a long time and is very interested about it all. She is very keen on babies.

A girl, 19 months :

From ten months old I haven't been able to get her to use it as she should do, and she has refused to sit on it, as soon as I have attempted to do so. This last week or so she has consented to sit on it, but it seems as if as soon as she does that it prevents her from passing anything, because as soon as she gets up she will do it by the side of it. I have tried talking to her, but without success. When I can see she wants to use it I quietly draw her to it or bring it to her, but she holds herself stiff and refuses to sit down.

A girl, 2½ years :

During the last week she will not sit down, for big or little duties, but holds it back until she does it in her knickers. She has not been scolded for it. Nanny has to give her oil and medicine each night, although she is not in the least constipated, and then it is two or three days before she does it, and then we had to use a suppository, and it is the same with her little duty. She will go all day without doing it, and in consequence is miserable, saying that her " seaty " hurts and that she wants to sit down, but cries when the chamber is produced and will not do anything. Already she is looking " washed out ".

My boy baby, aged 13 months, is rather a difficult child. In the nursing home they used to say ruefully he was born grumbling—and I must say he never was the sunny nature the elder girl was. He progressed normally until about 2 months, when he began to develop boils and eczema. His nurse kept him on the wrong diet, so I changed, and the next nurse brought him on till he was an entirely different baby. He always was a screamer and possessed unusual vocal power—amazing in a baby. At first, of course, it was the inadequate feeding and then the boils. But now he is exceedingly strong and big. And very healthy indeed. The trouble is that the moment he catches sight of the " throne " he simply begins to bawl and refuses completely to do what is required, even to the point of defying us for an hour together when we all know that he must want to be clean very badly indeed ; but he keeps it back and back—and there can be no trouble physically because immediately afterwards he presents us with a dirty nappy. All this is accompanied by shrieks of pure rage. We have tried persuading him, coaxing, leaving him alone to do his " duty ", suggestion, and every type of " throne " to meet with the situation. He has worn out three nurses who simply can't compete with the noise and temper, and we are dreadfully worried because we don't want to " break " his temper, yet one *must* cure his temper, which is really violent. He absolutely kicks and hammers on the " throne " table with anger and not a tear on his face. He started on the usual " pot ". Then he could not be left by himself, even secured to a chair, as he kicked it from beneath him. We therefore made him a wooden polished square seat to cover it. He then kicked the throne one way and the pot the other, levering himself by the bedpost. We then mounted it on a sort of platform which by his own weight was unable to be moved. He then moved sideways and covered himself with the contents of the pot. Finally we made arms and a back to it and a movable tray in front of him which, when fixed, prevents him from getting his hands inside. His fury when he beheld this was almost funny. He now puts the energy he exerted physically before into his roars.

My little boy is two and a half, and is on the whole forward for his age; is happy in his relations with other children. He himself is so far an only child. At about 14 months he declined to use his pot at all. Before he was two I tried again. Soon after he was two he was dry in the daytime; he, however, never used it for his " big ", which he seemed to prefer to do when alone in his room or in the garden. I never scolded him for this and he has never been smacked. When he was 2¼ I had a miscarriage and was in bed for ten days; it upset him rather at the time. After this he still did not use his pot, but took to doing it every other day only, and if I was on the spot and pulled his trousers down he would do it on the floor, then watch me clear it up into the pot, when he would empty it himself down the lavatory. Lately he has been going three days without a motion. He just refuses to let himself do it, and when he has at last done it, he says doubtfully, " It's not nasty, is it ? " A few days ago, a little girl he often plays with performed very nicely on her pot, but when she got up my little boy who was watching retched violently and was almost sick. On the fourth day I have felt obliged to use a soap stick to induce him to pass his motion. Of course he loathed it, and the result is that he is now simply miserable about the whole business. There is only one thing more that might have bearing on the matter, that is that about a week before Xmas he was sick twice in the night (I think this was with excitement), and after this he used to say when he went to bed, " I don't want to do any more sick ", and of course

I said, " No, we don't want any more sick." But he now says, " I don't want to do any ' big pot '," in just the same voice, and doubtless thinks it equally disgusting, though I have never consciously implied that either was objectionable as matter.

I have a little kiddicraft chair for my little boy (one year and nine months) and have tried my hardest to get him to use it, but with no avail, he is most intelligent over everything else. . . . After spending quite a time in the morning sitting him on the chair without success, he will do his business immediately I have put on his knickers. I have therefore given up the chair for a period, hoping time will improve matters. He still goes without any warning to me whatever, and then stands all huddled up crying, " Bizzy, Bizzy ", until I take it out ; he holds himself almost rigid, so that I have quite a job to remove his knickers. I have tried putting it in his little pot to let him see what it is for, but he refuses to look at it, and hides his head in my lap. . . . I had no trouble with him when a baby, and had no dirty nappies ; I might say I used to hold him out, not sit him on a pot, but when he was too heavy to hold I started to sit him on a little pot, when this trouble began. I have been most careful not to scold him in any way.

These quotations may suffice to show how urgent and difficult the situation may be to the child himself. We already know that it is so from the point of view of the mother, but what I am wanting to make clear is the intense feelings which the child shows about the request we make to him to defæcate or urinate at a given time and place, and about his inability to do so. Why does he show this apparent unreason and contrariness, this unshakable obstinacy

or great anxiety ? Why cannot he see how much
more simple and convenient it is if he will function
where and when we wish ? What is it that is so
puzzling and difficult for him, and that leads him to
resist persuading, coaxing, commanding, reproach-
ing, and punishing ?

We have learnt the answer to these questions, first
of all through the psycho-analysis of adults, who
have been enabled to recall or live again through
these early emotions and bewilderments ; more
recently, from the analysis of quite young children
at the very time when they were passing through this
phase of development. We have learnt that all
these bodily processes are of the utmost psychical
significance, and carry with them profound unconscious fantasies, concerned with the child's
relation to his mother and his mother's to him.
Ordinary observation of children who are not
altogether inhibited in talk and play will often yield
confirmation of psycho-analytic findings in this
respect.

But before I speak of the unconscious fantasies
associated with these difficulties, I would like to
point out how complex a problem the child has to
deal with even on the bodily side. He has to
acquire a technical skill, the difficulty and complexity of which we constantly underestimate. In
the earliest days of his life, the child's sphincters are
relatively relaxed. Later on they acquire more
muscular tone and are normally contracted, relaxing
again under the stimulus of the internal pressure of
urine and fæces ; and presently, this internal pressure is co-ordinated with the stimulus of contact or

temperature, or of a particular position of the body
when held by the mother. The child first has to
learn to retain the contents of the bladder or the
bowel, even perhaps under considerable internal
pressure, and then to relax this muscular control at
a particular time and place. This balance of con-
traction and relaxation in response to the time and
place and the demands of his mother involves the
mastery of highly complex co-ordinations; and it
would very often seem that the child's concern to
retain the contents of bladder or bowel makes him
unable to relax his muscles immediately on being
offered the appropriate time and place. Only later
does all this become relatively automatic. But in
addition to the problem of co-ordinating a complex
muscular system with internal conditions and with
the externally perceived situation, there is the position of the body as a whole to be considered. In
the beginning we usually give the child plenty of
support or actually hold him over the vessel. At a
certain age, however, sometimes very soon after the
child has gained a precarious balance of his body
and a rudimentary power of walking, we expect him
to balance his body on an uncomfortable rim of a
vessel (itself often too high), and to support his
general equilibrium without external aid at the same
time as he has to make this complicated co-ordination of inner and outer muscles. We are thus
demanding of him a highly complex co-ordination
of posture and of tension of particular parts, with
freedom and relaxation of the sphincters. We
usually ask him to achieve this on a moment's
demand, and, as I said, at a time when his general

bodily poise and control is extremely uncertain. It would surely be astonishing if he could achieve it all as easily as we expect and at the ages which we have somehow come to expect it, even apart from the more purely psychical problem. On bodily grounds alone, it is clear that we need to give the child every aid in learning to acquire this skill, and plenty of time for the skill to mature. Every detail with regard to size and position of the vessel, the support which we give him for general bodily balance, the ease of sitting down or standing up, will affect his mental attitude to the problem, and we ought not to demand this skill before the child is old enough to master it without difficulty.

To turn now to the meaning of the situation for the child's mental life. I have not time to give you a systematic account of the unconscious fantasies of the child connected with excretory processes. We have learnt what a wealth of such fantasies there is, and how varied and individual they can be, according to the previous history of the child and the way in which he has been handled by mother and nurse. There are certain general attitudes which every child shows at different phases of his development. Even these, however, are too complex and too rich in detail for me to be able to describe. All I can do is to mention some of his fantasies in order to make clear the point that these bodily processes have a mental significance for the child. They are instruments for expressing his emotions in relation to his mother and father; and his emotions are in their turn bound up with wishes and ideas that are not conscious, and that cannot be made so without the special procedure of psycho-analysis. But through this technique, we have learnt much about these ideas and wishes and the part they play in the developing ego of the child.

Observation of the earliest days of infancy suggests that in the beginning the process of defæcation is on the whole disagreeable, and we know that wind and colic pains occur very early in the life of the infant. Bowel movements are thus readily associated with pain or disagreeable tension, and this is one of the ways in which the contents of the bowel comes to be felt as a " bad " thing. After the second or the third months, however, when the necessary movements become better co-ordinated, there are plenty of signs that the infant finds the process of defæcation on the whole pleasurable, and since, like urination, it is generally associated with the most pleasurable experience of life in these early months, namely, taking in food at the mother's breast, there is a considerable period of development under favourable conditions when the excretory products are felt by the child to be as pleasant and good as the food taken in. At this time the baby feels that he is giving his mother urine and fæces in return for the milk which she is giving him. This attitude is most important for later development in love and trust, and one that we should do everything to foster by our handling and mode of expression. But for various reasons this picture is rarely sustained in the child without some disturbance. If the stool becomes solid, it will give some degree of pain in passing, and thus comes to be felt as a cutting, piercing instrument rather like the teeth. The child's problem with regard to his own development and his wish to bite is, as Mrs. Klein has shown you, of central significance for his emotional life and his later development, and since fæces often become identified with cutting, piercing teeth, this strengthens the feeling that they too are dangerous. Moreover, the child's biting wishes and the fantasies to which these wishes give rise lead him presently to regard the contents of his bowels, particularly the ejected contents, as the result of having bitten up his mother's breast—indeed, in fantasy, his whole mother. They are therefore dead, decaying, poisonous black stuff. They are dead, but since they move in the bowels and frequently hurt, they are not inert but actively malignant.

Moreover, the child in his own anger and aggression towards his mother wants to use these substances to attack and poison her with. From being the means of attack they then become in his unconscious fantasy identified with his own sadistic impulses, the " bad " part of himself. And then he wants all the more to get rid of them, the poisonous substances and the bad wishes alike; by putting the badness and the danger into someone else he projects them outside himself; and so he dirties the floor in such a way as to make his mother angry. He does this not out of a mere whim, but under this feeling of necessity to put this " badness " into someone else and get rid of it from himself. Whilst he is under the stress of these feelings and fantasies, he cannot easily come to learn that bringing these substances out and putting them in a particular place may be an act of love towards his mother.

We have, of course, to remember that we do in fact treat fæces and urine as " bad " by throwing them away. We do not preserve them and treasure them as we do our household goods or the child's toys. We put them down the drain and make them disappear as quickly as we can. The little child very often feels chagrin at this reception of his products, which constantly confirms his own notion of their " badness ". Moreover, the dark bowel product becomes linked up in his mind with all sorts of dark or black things which for other reasons are unpleasant or dangerous. For example, the blackness of grubby feet and fingers that people scold you for; the dark frown and flush of anger on the faces of people when you've done wrong, or been angry or bitten anyone; the black of a bruise, the black night that comes over your eyes like a blanket when the light is put out or when you shut your eyes; the black pupil of the eye, which seems to suggest that the whole of the inside of the body is black since you can see black through people's eyes; the black thunder-clouds that cover up the sun and make frightening noises and flooding rain. All this blackness and darkness and grubbiness is terrifying to the child when he is in a suspicious or hostile or frightened mood. In this and other ways the child comes to feel that the bowel products are bad and dangerous things which should be kept inside and not brought out openly. The discipline of the chamber-pot takes no reckoning of this significance of the fæces and urine, and of their dirtiness and dangerousness in the child's imagination. The child himself, however, because the pot is nice and

146

clean, hesitates to put into it something which he regards as foul. It is better by far to keep the whole thing hidden in the bed or in his knickers. Besides, there is not quite the same element of deliberation about defæcating in the bed or in his clothes. It just happens, it does not have to be thought about, it is effortless. Whereas this deliberate soiling of a nice clean pot is a desecration. No nice thing must be soiled or badly treated. Mother must not be. And yet she wants him to defæcate into this pot. But *he* wants to keep it clean, just as with his loving feelings he wants to save his mother from being bitten and dirtied. The fact that we prefer him to soil the pot rather than the napkin does eventually come home to him, but it cannot at first seem true or desirable, since he is under the domination of intense feelings connected with the fears of dirtying or poisoning, or in some way damaging his mother. In the unconscious layers of the mind, the child's fantasies refer to his acts towards his mother. All his bodily processes are connected with these fantasies about the person of his mother, since his own first relation to her (in suckling) was a bodily one. There is the additional factor that the mother herself takes an active interest in this particular bodily process. Hiding these substances is thus one way of denying them, and denying the unconscious intentions they convey. The child can pretend to himself that he has not got them there inside, whereas when he puts them in a pot, he sees and shows to others the unmistakable evidence of the damage he has done. The child's obstinate constipation and refusal to use the vessel

may therefore be an expression, not only of naughtiness and destructiveness, but also of his very wish
to be clean and to save his mother, indeed the whole
world, from coming into contact with the bad stuff
that he is keeping inside.

Another trouble is that a child (whether boy or
girl) in the early years may have a feeling of complete despair at the fact that he can *only* produce
these rejected substances from the body. He cannot have babies, or breasts which give good milk
like his mother, or a fertilizing penis like the father.
He does not yet even know how to make things
clean. All he knows is how to be dirty, and all he
can produce is dirtying substances. The tiny child
has so little experience to justify a belief in the
future. He does not know in any vital sense that
he will grow up and become able to have a baby or
to give one to a loved woman. All he knows is
that his father and mother can do these things, and
he can only produce substances that are thrown
away as "no good". When we become too
anxious about his constipation and try all sorts of
desperate remedies to compel him to yield up his
stool, we are of course confirming him in his belief
that the substance of his bowels is bad, since we
show him how worried we are if he keeps it inside
him. Perhaps the actual experience of congestion
and tension and temperature, and of course of the
pain of passing a large stool, help to confirm these
fantasies of the child.

In the same way the child has a wealth of fantasies
with regard to urine. This is another means of
expressing rage and fury with his mother when he

cannot get what he wants, it is another instrument of aggressive attack upon her. In his unconscious fantasy, he wishes to wet and drown and burn his mother with his urine—although at other times he may feel it to be a good gift towards her, given in return for her milk. In actual reality he finds that he can control her behaviour by his urine. He can make her frown with anger by his wetting and can give her endless trouble. When, later, he finds that thunderstorms and real rivers drown and damage people these seem to him to express his own magical fantasies of being able to do tremendous things with his own stream of urine. The heat of the urine, as well as of the excited genital, lead him to connect the urinary process with fire and burning as well as with wetting and urine. The uncontrollability of the need to urinate in the early months, like the involuntary movement of the bowels, is itself a source of anxiety about the uncontrollable things inside, the difficulty of controlling one's biting impulses and dirtying impulses and aggression and greed and hate.

Perhaps these details will serve to illustrate the general point that excretory processes and products are charged with the utmost personal significance for the child. They mean things he can do in hate and anger to the persons whom he also loves. The dangers which they carry are not built upon adult reality, the actual degree of inconvenience to the mother, but upon the ignorance and inexperience of the infant, as well as his irresistible wishes and over-whelming anxieties. I might, perhaps, as a final illustration of the meaning of these things to the child, quote a part of the analysis of one small boy.

X., aged four, was an ordinary, healthy, happy child, save for inexplicable fits of tantrums every now and then. Analysis showed many fantasies with regard to excremental processes. The child's father was dead. Fæces for him represented the dead and decaying father who had in fantasy been eaten up and bitten to pieces. The child felt himself to be full of black stuff from his hair to his toes. In his tantrums and violent screams he was trying to get rid of the dangerous black stuff inside him. The black stuff was indeed *identified* with his screams, since his screams make other people's faces go black in fury. His grandmother had recently had an operation on the eyes for cataract. The child showed quite plainly that he believed this blindness to be due to the black stuff which had come out of him, both through the bowel and through the mouth in screaming, and was equated with the darkness and the black night, and therefore with the blackness when one's eyes were closed and blind. When he had played in the garden and messed himself up with the soil, he was called a " gutter urchin ", and he showed me in analysis that this meant to him that he was so bad and dirty that he deserved only to be washed away down the drain of the w.c. ; in order to save his mother from temper and pain and his Granny from being blind, he ought to die.

But black things are not *only* " bad " to him, for he and his aunt and mother are devoted to a song by a black man about love : " They asked me how

I knew my own true love was true " and " something inside which I cannot hide, which cannot be denied ". X. has seen a film of little black boys swimming and enjoying themselves, wearing only loin cloths. He has been told that it is good to wear few or no clothes, because the sun makes one brown and strong and well. His logic runs, therefore, something like this : " If the black (or brown) is on the *outside* instead of being hidden inside as it is with me, if it is on the outside as it is with the black boys, who swim about and are so happy in the warm countries where there is no need to wear clothes, and may sun-bathe all day long and get strong and well, and learn how to sing these songs which mothers and aunts treasure so much, then everything is all right. Therefore it is better to *be* a black boy, and take every opportunity of soiling my legs and arms and face, since open dirtying is obviously less dangerous than hidden and secret dirtying." And as a consequence of this unconscious train of thought the boy did compulsively dirty himself in every possible way, both in the analytic room, and (in spite of protests and reproaches) in his home and garden. His need to do this lessened very considerably with the course of the analysis, as he came to understand what the fears were which compelled him to dirty himself, and how little these had to do with real things.

The precise meanings of a little child's behaviour about being clean or dirty will vary with the strength of his own feelings and with his personal history, but there will always be some intense emotions and inarticulate imaginings behind these difficulties.

III.   I am sure that what is in your minds now is the question of how the child gets over these acute crises; and especially what the best way is of helping him out of them.   Let us consider what happens in the minds of children who acquire a mastery of their functions easily, and are regular, clean and orderly in their bodily habits within the first three or four years.   In the first place, if the child has the ordinary opportunities for bodily movement, running and jumping and climbing, crawling, swinging and balancing, throwing and kicking, he becomes more and more secure in the poise and control of his body.   The purely technical problem of raising and lowering his body in an appropriate position, keeping some muscles taut and relaxing others at the right time, thus becomes easier and easier for him, and as it becomes easier it becomes less frightening.   As he grows more secure in this skill he is less afraid of falling into the pot, or of not being able to get up again from it, or of falling down the drain.   And all this comes as the result of time and growth, and of experience. No amount of exhortation or pleading will give the child of eighteen months or two years the skill normally attained by the child of three or four.   We can keep him from becoming skilful by giving him too little chance of practising movement and equilibrium, or by frightening him so that he gives up making an effort, and loses that sense of self-confidence which so greatly assists the beginner in the attainment of skill.   But we cannot force skill to appear, or accelerate the natural growth of nervous co-ordinations.   On this ground alone, therefore, patience and cheerful belief in the future is the best aid to mother and child.

This process of growth, and ripening of inherent abilities has, moreover, to be allowed for on the psychological side as well as the purely physical. No matter what we say or do we cannot produce in the child of two the developed sense of reality about the use of the pot, for example, or the developed understanding of our values and standards, which the child of four or five can and does attain under good conditions. We can aid or hinder this growth in natural balance of feelings, but we cannot force it to appear before the time is ripe. Moreover, there is a good deal of reason to think that this natural maturing of feelings and skills with regard to excretory processes will come about in the child, in an atmosphere of love and trust amongst clean and orderly adults, even without any specific teaching or training. After all, human beings are not the only clean animals. Many of the other animals are as particular as we are in this matter, and we cannot doubt that there is a natural tendency towards orderly behaviour in this respect. Moreover, the child learns not only by direct exhortation, but by all that he sees us do and say, and all that he absorbs of our feelings and values by watching and listening and responding to our moods. So that we have far more ground for trust in the future, even apart from explicit teaching on this matter, than most people seem to realize. If he lives amongst clean people who are loving and understanding, as well as clean, the child will become clean and orderly like them; and he will do this far more readily and with far less difficulty on the way if no attempt is made to force this skill upon him before he is ripe to achieve it. His identification with adults who are friendly and understanding as well as clean is one of the fundamental processes which leads him to be clean and orderly too.

In such a helpful atmosphere of encouraging love, the child learns that his fantasies about the harm that his bodily products may do are not based upon reality. He finds that the pot is not harmed because he deposits " bad " stuff in it. It can be made clean again and with very little trouble, much less trouble than when he soils his clothes or the bed. He learns that even if his mother is a little impatient with the trouble that he causes her, he does not actually poison or drown her or make her irreparably cruel and unforgiving. Every one of his fantasies comes under the control of real experience as he grows from infancy to later childhood. Furthermore, he makes the discovery of so many other ways in which he can express his need for power, and this most primitive bodily expression thus loses its attraction. There are other substances, sand and garden soil and mud, plasticine and clay, that he can play and make things with and even produce things that call out pleasure and interest from others. He can splash and pour with water in a way that does no harm to anybody. He can combine water and paint to daub and smear, and presently to produce pictures in colour and form, that give delight to him and others. He can build with bricks and dig in the garden to make plants grow, and in endless ways his fingers can learn to express the feelings and fantasies primarily connected with the sphincter muscles and the bodily substances. This displacement of interest from bodily parts and products to external objects and skills gradually releases the physiological organs for physiological functions, and reduces their importance as organs of pleasure and comfort. The child's creative interests in the outside would become not only a substitute for primitive pleasure, but the best reassurance against primitive anxieties.

All these processes, the natural ripening of bodily skill and emotional balance, the tempering of fantasies by real experience, the acquisition of the creative arts, and identification with his parents, are going on together ; and then presently they enable the child to achieve a normal orderly functioning of the primitive bodily processes with a minimum of disturbance and difficulty. And this functioning gradually becomes more or less automatic. A habit is thus in the end achieved, but later than most of the text-books suppose ; and it is achieved, not by early reflex conditioning, but as the outcome of a long and complex psychological development.

Let us now consider what the psycho-analyst can suggest as to the best way of helping the child through this long process to skilful achievement.

In the first place, it is important not to imagine that there is any method that will solve all the child's difficulties in a moment. Most of these difficulties are to a greater or less extent inherent in the human situation. They cannot be altogether avoided, no matter what we do. Moreover, the child's feelings are so obscure to himself that it is not surprising that mother and nurse cannot quite understand them, with the best will in the world. There is, therefore, no need for us to feel such intense shame and guilt because the child suffers temporary unhappiness about his bodily processes, or because he is somewhat later than the majority of children in becoming clean. We are not omnipotent, and must not blame ourselves for not being so.

Secondly, it is helpful to remember at every point that the sphincter muscles of bladder and bowel do not function as a simple local mechanism, and that we cannot act upon these in any simple way uncomplicated by the child's feelings about us. Whatever we do or say to the child, we are always dealing with a whole human being, and with his active emotions of love and hate, of trust and fear. These bodily processes are part of his emotional expression towards other people ; if we remember this, we are not so likely to act in a way which the child himself feels to be an outrage, or which terrifies him with a sense of failure and weakness. The question of suppositories is one case in point. There may be times when enemas and suppositories are necessary on strictly *medical* grounds ; but these times are far rarer than most people realize, and it has to be recognized that when they need to be given for reasons of bodily health, they are nevertheless always undesirable psychologically, since the child feels that the physical interference is an attack upon his body. In addition, the enema or suppository increases the sense of helplessness from which so many of the child's difficulties arise, because he feels that he has lost control over the objects in his body ; and his fear of grown-ups as ruthless avengers for his naughtiness and guilt is thus augmented. To give suppositories and enemas as an *educational* means is wholly to be condemned. These things do not educate the normal voluntary functioning of the sphincter muscles. They retard it, invariably increasing the tendency to constipation.

The facts I have quoted as to the frequency of breakdowns after the end of the first year in apparently well-established habits offer clear evidence that it is a waste of time and effort to give too much attention to the forming of early reflex habits. But we can go much further than this, and say that too early a start is definitely undesirable, since it raises expectations in the mother that cannot be sustained, and tends to increase the child's anxiety about the whole process. You will remember that Mrs. Klein suggested that training in cleanliness should not coincide with weaning. I see no particular harm in getting the child to use the pot in the early days for one's own convenience, provided that no special importance is attached to it from the child's point of view, and no disappointment is felt when the child fails to make use of it. The early response of the child to the stimulus of the pot bears little if any relation to his real problem of acquiring voluntary control later, when his awareness of this process as a means of pleasing or annoying his mother has developed. Quite a large number of children, both here and in other countries, with whom no attempt is made to train so early to the pot, at fifteen or eighteen months gain skill and security with practically no trouble at all. It would not surprise me if a wide study of comparative evidence on this point showed that the children with whom no pot training had been done before the first or second quarter of the second year actually took to it then with much less anxiety and disturbance than those who had been brought up on it. This may of course be because the mothers and nurses have not had unjustified expectations, and therefore not felt disappointment and shame. They could then handle the child at the time when they did begin training him with much more confidence and gentleness. There is not much doubt that the mother's attitude in this relation is quite as important as the child's.

When once training has begun, there is no doubt that regular opportunities are helpful, for example with regard to evacuation of the bowels. But contrary to the general view, regularity should not be overstressed. Some people cling to the idea that the child *must* empty his bowels at a particular time every day, almost as if this were a religious axiom. I do not believe this to be a wise attitude. We can overdo our prying into the child's bowel processes, and conjuring up in his mind pictures of terrible internal dangers if he does not empty his bowels at a particular hour every morning. The child is more likely to function in an easy and natural way, according to the general needs of his body, if he is not terrified about the whole thing by having impressed upon him the great evils of not evacuating at a particular time. In general, one can say that too great insistence upon these processes from any point of view is hampering. Too much emotion in the mind of the mother stirs up too much feeling in the child's mind, and it is so easy, by our own show of anxiety and insistence upon immediate action, to confirm the child's spontaneous fantasies about the awful dangers of the bowel contents and bowel action. Moreover, if we are too insistent, we not only compel the child to defend himself against our ruthless interference with his insides by withholding the stool, but give him a very powerful weapon for tyrannizing over us in his turn. All these attitudes are fairly certain to produce a costive tendency. It is far more helpful to convey to the child that the process is a natural and a good one and that the body can be trusted to act for its own good.

Along with this goes the question of terminology. One could find many children whose only words for these organs and processes are negative terms, implying something bad or shameful. One little boy, for example, has no other word for his genital than " rudy ", and no other way of expressing his need to urinate than saying, " I want to be excused." The ordinary nursery terms that arise from the child's first vocalizations about these processes are far better than adult words expressing shame and disgust.

If one begins training somewhere in the first half of the second year, how early can one expect full control to be achieved? The answer to this is obviously to be found in the comparative study of large numbers of children. It is now pretty gener- ally agreed that under favourable conditions, that is in nurseries where regular opportunities are given in a friendly and helpful way, the control of the bowels is commonly achieved at about eighteen months and that of the bladder in the daytime at about two years. Many children, however, are later than this. These figures are only rough general norms, the chief value of which is to prevent us from putting our expectations too high. It is true that some children will be clean earlier than this, but we have no ground for *demanding* it from any child. You will see then how unwise it is to talk about " leaving off the nappies at seven to eight months ", and how unjustified is the despair of the many mothers who say that a child of fourteen or sixteen months is " shamefully dirty ". Many perfectly normal and happy children will not achieve success until a good deal later than eighteen months and two years. Night-time dryness is in any case a good deal later than daytime. How many miseries and heart-burnings would be saved if mothers realized that it is quite common for children to wet their beds in their third years or even their fourth! " Surely at her age she should be clean," has been said to me about children of ten or thirteen months ! One mother of a child of ten months said, " It is dreadful to be beaten by one so young." We really have no right to say that a child *should* be clean at a certain age. I often wish that the books supposed to help mothers and nurses in training their children would not say the child " should be " clean at a certain age, but content themselves with stating that many children if properly helped are clean at, say, eighteen months or two years. There is no need to feel shame and despair about a child whose difficulties are a little more acute than the average, since he, too, will grow through them if the mother's attitude is patient and encouraging.

It is true that by laying too much stress upon the matter, we may sometimes terrify the child into being clean ; but we are very liable to start up other more serious difficulties. A striking case of this was reported to me recently. A boy of two and a half, a happy, healthy, well-developed child, lost the nurse whom he had had from birth, and who had tended and trained him with love and understanding. His only fault at this age was that he still wetted his bed once each night, but he had been clean and dry in the daytime for some time. The nurse left to be married, and her loss was a very great one to the child. The new nurse, less sympathetic and understanding, was extremely shocked at discovering a boy of two and a half years who wet his bed in the night, and made it her one concern that the child should give up this bad habit. She woke the boy every hour during the night to make him use the pot, and expressed shame and disgust at his dirtiness. At the end of six weeks the boy was perfectly dry by night as well as by day, but he was so terrified of not being clean that he was waking at all hours of the night in great anxiety, and running to the w.c. every few minutes during the day. And he had developed a bad stammer. The nurse had gained her end—but at what a cost ! This is quite a common sort of happening when the mother or the nurse makes a sudden determined attempt to cure the child's dirtiness in a hurry, and I could give many other such dramatic instances of a tragic interference with the child's normal development towards cleanliness. One little girl of three was so severely scolded by a nurse for a single wetting that she refused to urinate for twenty-seven hours, until the mother was in despair.

What I have said about the technical problem of bodily skill for the child in learning to use the chamber-pot successfully, and the fears and fantasies connected with this, will suggest to you the wisdom of giving him real ease and real support in his bodily position during the process. For some years now I have been recommending the use of the commode chair during the training to the use of the pot. The commode chair will not in itself work miracles and make the child clean if the general attitude of the mother and nurse is unfavourable, but it does help him to get over his fears of falling, and it makes real independence for him possible much earlier than the use of the bare pot (surely a clumsy and un-comfortable object !). Again, when it is desired to make the transition from the chair or pot to the lavatory seat, many mothers have found that the child can be greatly helped by the use of an extra seat with a smaller hole, which can be placed on top of the ordinary adult seat, and a firm foot-rest of some kind given to help the child to support his position without strain and anxiety.

In beginning training, it is advisable not merely to offer the pot to the child regularly at times when he is likely to need it, but also to watch for the signs of his needing it, the slight restlessness, the hand going to the genital, the appearance of distraction, a slight flush, or slight tension in the legs, and so on,

which we all learn to recognize. If, when it is clear
that the child has the urge to urinate or defæcate,
we then, with gentle, cheerful suggestion, show him
the appropriate place, we are far more likely to be
able to set up the habit of functioning in that place
than if we take no notice beforehand but merely
scold him after he has wet the floor or his garments.
Many mothers have found that this method worked
beautifully, so that the child was quite soon showing
signs of expectancy for the desired help of the
proffered pot along with the need to use it. When
we fail to seize the golden moment in this way, but
allow the child to wet and then scold him, he very
often fails to understand that we are scolding
him for soiling a particular place and feels quite
intensely that we are scolding him for the act of
urinating itself; or that we are expressing our disapproval of his having the substance in him. How
can the little child differentiate these feelings unless
we help him by making the situation as clear as
possible, and unless we encourage his understanding
by our friendliness? Fear always inhibits the child's
intelligence, so that he is bound to be slower in
learning if we scold and reproach than if we show
him precisely what we want him to learn in a clear
but friendly way.

A great many children learn habits of cleanliness,
or get over an acute phase of difficulty, far more
readily if things are arranged so that they can tend
themselves. The commode is one example of such
help. The child's clothes are another. If we make
these difficult for him to unfasten in time so that he
has to depend upon us for help, we are retarding

his development. As early as possible we should try to make his garments easy to undo or to slip down, so that he can fend for himself in this matter. With regard to training in the night, if we insist that he shall call for our attention after an age when he really could look after himself, we often increase his difficulties. If we arrange a small vessel, for example an enamel mug for a boy or a light and smallish enamel pot for a girl, in an easily accessible position near his bed, and as early as possible help him to learn to get out of bed and look after himself when the urge arises, calling for us if he is in difficulties, but not compelling him to waken us and to be handled in a helpless way, he will gain this night-time skill much more easily. All the details of garments and vessels and supports make a big difference to the child, not only through their technical aid or hindrance, but also because they express our essential attitudes to the child. If we put him in an uncomfortable position and then demand that he shall function, we are proving ourselves enemies of his growth and of his peace of mind. If we show that we understand the technical difficulties of the skill we want him to acquire, and are willing to help and to wait while he acquires it, he feels the love and understanding in this, and has far more confidence in us. The mother or nurse who once understands this will find specific ways of helping individual children which cannot be detailed in a general account. Perhaps an example will show what I mean. One mother told me that when her boy of fourteen or fifteen months, whom she was trying to train to the use of a pot on her knee, was held, no matter how firm and gently, with his back to her, he would only stiffen and scream and refuse to function. But if she held him facing her so that he could see her expression, and by putting his arms around her help himself actively to a secure position, he was happy and easy and functioned without any difficulty. This is an instance which serves to demonstrate beyond cavil the general truth I have tried here to make plain : that we are always con‑ cerned with the whole child and with his feelings towards us as human beings and helpers, not with a local mechanism.

This illustration also serves to show how children will differ in their feelings and their needs. Such idiosyncrasies need to be understood and to be respected—for example, one child will function best if left alone in the room on a comfortable seat ; another will be happier if mother or nurse stays near and speaks encouragingly. No single method will suit every child, but the mother or nurse who is not obsessed by the bogey of habit, and yet has trust in the child's growth, will easily be able to meet the particular needs of the particular child.

In general, we need a sense of proportion about this matter. The nurse I mentioned whose tactless behaviour brought on a stammer within six weeks of her taking charge obviously had no sense of pro‑ portion. It not seldom happens that mother or nurse feels the world will stand still unless the child is compelled to be clean at instant notice. Occa‑ sional breakdowns will occur with every child, under the stimulus of some important external event or some special phase of emotional development. If

we are able to understand that the young are really
only immature and unskilful, not wicked and per-
verse, when they cannot do all that we feel to be
right, and our plans appear to be going wrong, if
we have faith in the future and patience to wait for
the child's growth without misgiving, we shall not
readily imagine, if an accident should occur or a
period of difficulty ensue, that all our work has been
shattered at one blow.

To summarize these recommendations broadly :
in the first place, it is very important *not* to over-
emphasize habit, with regard either to early training
or later breakdowns, and not to take an over-simple
view of the child's problem in learning this complex
skill. Secondly, it is necessary to base our expectations upon reasonable standards, and to recognize
the individual rate of growth and the particular
emotional needs of each child. Nothing we can do
will prevent or remove all difficulties of development, just because the child is not a machine and we
are not omnipotent controllers of his destiny. But
time and the child's own natural ripening of skill
and emotional balance are on our side. If we give
him the appropriate physical aid and support, with
confident encouragement and a happy relation, he
will win safely and securely through these temporary
difficulties of growth.

VI. THE NURSERY AS A COMMUNITY

BY SUSAN ISAACS, C.B.E., M.A., D.SC.

THE title of this chapter might perhaps suggest that I am going to speak about " the nursery as a community " in the sense of a developed ideal, a philosophical or educational aim. I am not going to do this ; but, on the other hand, the purpose of this book as a whole might indeed be said to consider how far it is possible to approximate the nursery to a community in this ideal sense, one in which there is some definite plan controlling the behaviour of each member, father, mother, nurse, older and younger children, to each of the others, a plan in which their mutual actions and reactions are articulated according to a consciously desired end. You will remember what Miss Sharpe says about the implicit and explicit plans of parents, in Chapter I. Most of us have some plan for our children, of a varying degree of explicitness, arising from our own personal philosophy and personal loyalties, which in turn rest upon our own particular psychic equilibrium. We may desire, for instance, to promote the education of children in the nursery so that nursery life can be an adequate preparation for life in the school or in the adult world later on, or perhaps act as a corrective to the adult world as it exists at present. There are few who do not reflect upon the problem of how far the education of young children might contribute to solving the issues of war and peace, of economic maladjustment, or of personal responsibility under democracy.

It so happens that a large part of my own life is directly concerned with the education of little children, and as an educator, I have fairly definite notions about what I want the nursery to aim at being, purposes which rest upon many diverse considerations, besides the contributions of psychoanalytic knowledge. In this chapter, however, I am writing specifically as a psycho-analyst. You want to know what light psycho-analysis, with its unique knowledge of the unconscious mental life of the child, can throw upon the particular educational or social issues with which you are concerned, and what limits and controls this special knowledge may entail for our main educational purposes.

In the previous chapters, a number of particular educational problems have already been discussed. Mrs. Klein, for example, dealt with the technique of breast-feeding and weaning, Miss Searl with the answering of children's questions, Dr. Middlemore with the child's sensual life, and I myself with training in cleanliness. Psycho-analysts see reason to believe that if these various situations could be generally handled with a greater degree of wisdom than is commonly found to-day, a great deal of mental stress which in later life not only appears in personal conflict, but serves to augment social disruption and international strife, would be mitigated.

In this chapter I am going to deal not so much with specific issues as with the broader aspects of the relation between adults and children in the nursery, the problems of discipline and parental authority, and of the child's play with his fellows. I shall follow the method I adopted in discussing the problem of cleanliness. That is to say, I shall first of all consider the nature of the child's psychological relationships to other people, and then go on to discuss what educational use we can make of these facts, and how far they may limit and control or revivify our conscious aims.

I shall deal not only with those universal mental processes which we discover through analysis in every child, but shall also refer at many points to the specific influence of his particular parentage and real experiences upon the final outcome of the child's inherent mental tendencies. The real qualities of the parents make an enormous difference to the child's development, and the effect of their behaviour is never to be underestimated. And yet it is not in itself the whole problem. The child's inner psychic life has its own contribution to make to the complexity of his relation with his parents ; that is to say, we have not only to consider the behaviour of the parents from our point of view as experienced adults, but what it means to the child himself, with all his limitations of feeling, of understanding and of experience. Even with the best parents in the world, the most considerate and the most skilful, the child will have his internal prob-

lems, since these arise from the inherent issues of
human development. He will solve them with
far greater ease if his parents help him, but they
will be none the less real to him, just because he is a
child. It is the way in which the particular qualities of the parents and of the real environment inter-
act at every point with the child's own psychic
processes that is the question before us.

Let us consider, in the first instance, then, the
ordinary child of ordinary parents, who train him
according to the best that they understand. The
mother shows her affection by her patient care and
devotion. She baths and comforts him and ar-
ranges for quiet sleep and tends the child according
to the regular routine which is thought best for his
digestion and bodily growth. What difficulties,
then, can the child suffer in such a home ? Does
he not develop in complete comfort and mental
peace, resting upon an unqualified sense of the love
and devotion of his mother ? He certainly attains a
far greater degree of mental health and happiness
under these favourable conditions than if he is
starved and neglected or handled roughly, or-seri-
ously misunderstood—as we shall see in many details. And yet difficulties occur, even under these
favourable conditions. And they are much greater
than we naïvely assume, when we think only of the
objective care which his mother showers upon him.
From his side the picture is in many ways quite different. For his part, he knows hardly anything yet
of time and space and real events. When he is
hungry, he does not know that food is coming to
him presently. He cannot realize that his mother

has her eye on the clock and is making preparations even while he waits in frustrated pain. He comes to realize this later on, and to recognize all the signs of future satisfaction. But in the beginning his emotions are immediate and unqualified. Apart from times of sleep, he is either satisfied and blissful, sucking at the breast and feeling the pangs of hunger gradually stilled within him, or he is given up to unqualified, untempered wishes and the intense pain of their frustration. Whether it be satisfaction or loss, pain or pleasure, the infant's experience is absolute. He does not even know that his mother is there in the world as a source of future satisfaction, except when he touches her and takes her nipple into his mouth. Presently, he recognizes her existence through his eyes, and if his eyes can rest upon her, remains content that she is alive as the source of security and satisfaction ; but even now, she is not there when he does not see her. He has no guarantee that she will come back again when she is not visibly present. We know how, towards the end of the first year, he loves to play the game of " peek-a-boo ", and gets great pleasure from the disappearance and reappearance of the loved object. At this age he has got so far that he can play this game of loss and recovery ; but of course at nine or ten months he has travelled a very long way from the earliest days of infancy, and is already a highly sophisticated person. In the first three or four months he has no security except in immediate personal satisfaction, and his feelings are violent commensurably with the absoluteness of his experiences. When he has to wait, his inability to

bear frustration is shown in his rage and fury, in his
screaming and kicking, and, presently, in his biting
and scratching and wetting and dirtying.   Life for
the infant is thus felt as a series of " good " and
" bad " moments, which in the beginning are
largely separate experiences.   The " good " moments are almost identical with the " good "
mother who brings them, and with his own " good "
feelings of love and satisfaction when he receives
them.   On the other hand, the " bad " moments of
frustration and loss, and the child's own " bad "
feelings of rage and pain and fury, give rise to the
image of the " bad " mother, to whom all these
things are attributed.   Moreover, the " bad " con-
sists not only of hunger and oral cravings, but in
the first few weeks of such experiences as too bright
a light, too sudden a noise, a marked change of
temperature, a lump in his garments, indeed, all
those painful external stimuli which the infant's
psyche finds so hard to tolerate in the beginning.
The " good " mother not only suckles and satisfies
hunger and the need for love, but removes these too
bright lights or too loud noises and all the other
painful stimuli from the outer world.   This, then,
is the picture of the world and of himself as the
infant experiences these in the first two or three
months.   And he cannot yet know anything of his
mother's sense and control and the ordered knowledge and developed character in which he could
trust.   He knows only these isolated and distinct
high lights of experience.   His mother thus becomes " bad " to him whenever, for any reason, he
is kept waiting in hunger or in momentary discom-

fort. Just as he has no knowledge of the ordered way in which she serves him, so he has no knowledge of the reasons why she does not at this moment satisfy him. He knows nothing, for example, of her responsibilities to other children or to her husband or herself; and indeed he has no wish for such knowledge or such facts. He lives imperiously upon his need to have her for himself.

All this is the expression, first, of the child's compelling need to have his mother serve him, without which he could not survive, and secondly of his own lack of a developed ego, of any knowledge of time and space and ordered relations. He has as yet no past and no future, only the imperative present of intense feeling.

So much can be seen by empirical observation of the infant, without the special knowledge which the psycho-analytic study of the child's fantasy life has given us. By means of this special instrument, however, in the study of the dreams and fantasies of adults and the play of little children, we have gained a further piece of insight. In the beginning, the child not only sees his mother in the outside world as alternatively " bad " and " good ", now the one and now the other; but feels this " bad " and " good " mother also *within* him. He is a suckling, and takes his mother's nipple into his mouth and her milk into his body in the act of suckling. You know how much the mouth dominates the child's activity in these earliest months. His hand is for a long time the mere servant of the mouth, even when it becomes skilful in grasping and picking up external objects. Up to nine or ten months almost

173

everything that the child picks up is put into his mouth, since that is the source of his most vivid experiences, and his normal way of mastering and possessing the world. It is only after nine or ten months that the hand becomes an independent organ of mastery. His general attitude to the world at this time is essentially the desire to take outside things into his own body and his own mind. He " drinks in " and " absorbs " his mother's voice and face through his eyes and his ears and his own firm grasp, and thus builds up concrete pictures of his mother, whether satisfying or frustrating, within his own psyche. From the point of view of adult objective reality, we know that the mother remains outside the infant and independent of him, even though she suckles him at her breast, and even though he retains a living image of her in his memory and imagination. But from the point of view of the deepest and most primitive levels of psychic reality, the child actually feels his mother to be *inside* his mind, acting upon him there with all the qualities which he has seen or felt in her in the outside world, whether " good " or " bad ". The " good " mother of the moments of love and satisfaction is identified with the " good " substances and with feelings of warmth, comfort and well-being within his own body. And the " good " mother is greatly desired as an internal possession, since she is the ultimate source of well-being, both internal and external. In a similar way, the " bad " mother who frustrates him *in his fantasy* attacks him from within, eating him up as he has swallowed her in hunger or in rage ; wetting him, as in those urinary fantasies I have instanced he has wetted and drowned her. All the attacks which the child wants to make upon his mother in his bad moments of pain and fury, he now dreads that she will make upon him *from the inside*. And this " bad " fantasied mother inside him is identified with all the real experiences of internal processes, movements of the bowel, wind in the stomach, colic, pressure of fæces or urine ; and the difficulty of controlling bodily processes and substances is identified in the child's mind with the difficulty of controlling the " bad " parents inside.

These fantasies of internalized objects are not at all easy for us to understand, since they are so remote from ordinary adult reality. But they are of the utmost significance for the child's emotional problems. They form the deepest source of his tantrums and obstinacy, for example, or his feeding difficulties and tendency to dirtiness in the second and third years, as well as of his phobias and night terrors. And such fantasies underlie many of the normal activities of adults, too, in a way that I could make plain to you if time allowed. Let me remind you again that I am not speaking only of the unusual or abnormal child. These are the things that happen to every child, even the happiest.

Meanwhile, however, even in these earliest months, the development of the child's ego is also going on. The postural control of his own body, the co-ordination of hand and eye and ear and taste, and the consequent articulation of his perceptual world, are all developing apace. Round about five months, this seems to reach such a level that the child now becomes aware of his mother as a whole person, external and independent of himself. In the beginning she was to him little more than a breast to feed him and a pair of arms to enfold him. By about five months, however, he has woven into his perception of her as a whole all the sights and sounds and contacts of an endlessly varied kind which he has received from her in the course of her ministrations. He now sees her as the objective source of his life and love and satisfaction. Five months of age appears to be a quite critical time for development in a great many both intellectual and emotional ways, which I have not time to detail. In a recent paper which will prove to be a landmark in psychological science, Mrs. Klein[1] has shown us that the central problem of the child's whole life is faced at this period when he gradually becomes aware of his mother as a whole person. It is at this time that he first realizes that those primitive pictures of the " bad " mother and the " good " mother are not separate and distinct entities, but aspects of one and the same person, towards whom he, the child, feels these contrary impulses of love and hate. The " bad " mother is the mother whom he rages against in his fury and wants to destroy because she cannot satisfy him in the moment of demand. The " good " mother is she who feeds and tends and loves and makes him secure. But these are not in fact separate, they are one and indivisible. And this is his problem, his realization of the fact that his mother, his own real external mother, is the focus of his own intense and irre-

[1] " A Contribution to the Psycho-genesis of Manic-Depressive States," *Int. J. of Psycho-Analysis*, 1935, XVI, 145.

concilable feelings of love and of hate. This
awareness of his own conflicting feelings is intolerable to the child. It is indeed intolerable to us
adults also. It may happen that you have sufficient
self-awareness to know something of how painful
it is to realize that one hates a person whom one
loves, and has impulses of rage and destruction
against those whom one also values and treasures
and desires above all else. It is an intensely depress-
ing truth to have to face. The pain is hardly to be
borne, and it has to be lessened or got rid of by
some means. For the little child, this is the nodal
problem of his whole development. It is relatively
easy for the adult to control anger against those
whom he loves. In so far as we do not remain
under the domination of infantile modes of response,
we can learn to control and temper these impulses.
But the path from the earliest moment of this conflict between love and hate to adult reason and
moderation is a long one, traversing all the years
of the child's development. The whole story of
his growth could be stated in terms of his struggle
with this fundamental conflict. All the varied possibilities of later achievement in social life, of personal
skill and character, of neurosis or psychosis, have
their deepest source in this central issue.

There are as many individual modes of dealing
with this focal problem of development as there
are individual persons, and the particular flavour of
each of our personalities will always be related to
our special choice of ways out of this struggle.
Certain broad modes of response occur to a greater
or less extent in every one of us, however, and the

understanding of these broad mental processes throws light upon the general characteristics of the ordinary child's behaviour in the early years. Moreover, it is only in so far as we understand something of what this problem means to him that we can hope to plan our own behaviour to the child so as to help him forward in the direction of constructive achievement.

Let me now speak briefly of some of the more general modes of solution of this central problem typically shown by the ordinary child in the nursery. And let us look particularly at the ways in which he eventually achieves a more or less successful solution, carrying him forward on the path of personal achievement and of happy social relations with other people. I shall only have time to instance a few of these major mental attitudes, and my account will be far from systematic. My aim is to give you a sense of the complexity of the child's problem, in order to emphasize his need for the real help which we can give him, in the various directions I shall presently suggest.

One of the first ways in which the child tries to deal with this problem of loving and hating the same person is to reinstate the separateness of the " bad " mother and the " good " mother, " splitting " the unified perception of the whole mother into " bad " and " good " figures. This splitting of " bad " and " good ", and of the impulses and feelings towards the " bad " and " good " objects, is an enormously important mental process in ordinary adult life as well. It is happening in all of us whenever we believe that a particular person is wholly and entirely good, or another is wholly and entirely bad—our friends and our enemies, the hero and the villain, the saint and the criminal. These are diverse expressions of this primitive fantasy of the absolutely " good " and the absolutely " bad " mother. They do not correspond to reality, they are crystallizations of those absolute modes of feeling and of experience belonging to our earliest days. In the little child's behaviour, this process of splitting is often shown in the way he seeks help and protection and love from one person whilst flying in fear and distress from another. It is a common nursery situation for a child of, say, two years or more, who is quiet and docile with either nurse or mother alone, to become querulous and defiant if both nurse and mother are present. This puzzling behaviour arises in part from the fact that the child is struggling with his own love and hate for each person by separating these impulses, turning the love wholly in one direction and the hate wholly in another (whether it be mother and nurse, or mother and father). In this way he relieves his own internal tension, and very often he actually receives more love from the one person and more hate from the other, as a result. The nurse upon whom he turns his back naturally finds it hard to remain pleasant and calm in the face of rejection ; the mother is tempted into petting and consoling him when he turns to her. And this, we must realize, is the very situation which the child is trying to establish, partly because he feels more justified in his spitefulness against his nurse if she is less agreeable to him. Many little children are extraordinarily acute in their discernment of the ways in which they can produce a rift between the parents or between mother and nurse. The child can only remain loving to two people together when his development has made it possible for him to tolerate more of his own aggressive impulses towards a loved person, when he thus has less need to separate the " bad " and the " good " in himself and in others. He has then more confidence in his power to control the " bad " by means of the " good ".

The child's wish to separate any two grown-ups whom he sees together does not of course arise only from his need to separate his own impulses of love and hate and the internal " bad " and " good " mothers. In large part also it springs from his straightforward love and jealousy. He wants to be first in the affections of his mother and turn the nurse or the father out from this desirable position. He cannot bear to be left out in the cold while they love each other.

The child's early relations with his mother and father are thus very complicated. In the beginning, of course, the mother dominates the child's world entirely, but even in the second half of the first year, and typically in the second to the fourth years, the child finds his father attractive also and seeks love from him. This turning to the father, however, is not only to a person who is loved for his own sake. Since his mother was inevitably the first source of frustration as well as satisfaction and, therefore, the first object of his rage, the child presently, to some extent, turns away from her and seeks his father as a person who has not yet inflicted disappointments and frustrations, and has not yet been attacked in anger.

With those children who are in fact well treated, and with whom there is no untoward circumstance, this turning to the father does not have to be a turning from the mother, save in a relative and temporary degree. But sometimes this does happen, either because the mother is not in fact wise and loving, or because in some way she cannot give the child the satisfaction he needs, thus becoming to him almost entirely an object of disappointment and pain, and therefore of anxiety. He then turns away from her completely to look for some helper with a compensating degree of good, someone who can better satisfy his need for love. The great *dependence* of very young children upon a ministering adult is partly the result of this need for perfectly good and helpful grown-ups to counter all the memories of pain and frustration, and above all, to counter the fantasied " bad " mother inside the child's own mind.

The child's first natural feelings of rivalry with one parent for the love of another are thus strongly reinforced by the process of splitting of the " good " and the " bad ". The child must have one of the parents as a helper in order to fend off his fear of the other. Sometimes he has to swing about rapidly in his allegiances, from one parent to another, because each in turn (he imagines) becomes damaged and destroyed through his renewed needs and rages.

A little later the child's anxiety about his earliest aggressions is deflected anew into the conflicts he experiences with regard to other children. I am sure I do not need to take time in giving you evidence about the frequency and intensity of the tiny child's jealousy with regard to the new baby or a visiting child. I need only concern myself to show how this jealousy too is deeply reinforced by this nodal conflict of feelings towards his mother. His jealousy is so great and bitter partly because he feels the presence of the new baby to be the proof of his own unlovableness, or a punishment for his own naughtiness towards her, as well as because of his direct longing to be the centre of love, and his direct sense of loss and frustration. On the other hand, the child often also gains great comfort from the arrival of another child, since it is the surest proof that his own real or fantasied aggression has not done unlimited damage to his mother or finally separated her from his father. The new baby may at first stir up fresh sources of anger and hatred, but it is in the end also a new source of love and pleasure for the child, as well as a great reassurance about his anxieties that he has damaged and spoilt the life and the love within his mother.

You will find the same process going on with regard to toys and playthings. The little child will often want to break to pieces or to throw away any of his possessions which he has damaged. If he has hurt a thing it must be treated as altogether bad and got rid of, because he does not then feel so keenly the pain of having spoilt something that he values. He can turn to a new object with the assurance that it is entirely unharmed and therefore to be only loved. The ready " boredom " that many children show with toys which they have had for only a short time is an expression of this anxiety about spoiling things. As soon as one has used them, they become dirty, spoilt or damaged, and the dirty or damaged object seems to reproach one, so it is better to treat it as altogether bad, and turn away to a new one for fresh satisfactions.

I spoke just now of the relief which the child gains in being angry with one adult when there is another near by to act as helper. There is another source of comfort to him in this situation, in that he is able to project on to the nurse from whom he turns away those bad feelings of his own which cause him so much distress. In clinging to his mother against the nurse, he behaves as if he were saying to his mother, " It is she, my nurse, who is bad, not I. You and I can be good together if only she is turned out."

Now this process of *projection* is an enormously important one, not only in the life of the little child, and in the life of the insane adult, who deals with his own aggression by believing that all the world is plotting to murder him. It is scarcely less significant in many aspects of international life— for example, the hatred of political enemies, or the attribution of all disasters and difficulties to the machinations of a particular group of people— capitalists, socialists, communists, Jews, Germans, Japanese, Abyssinians. In all these feelings and beliefs, we see at work the insidious process of projecting on to an outside object the abhorred tendencies within oneself. Examples of this behaviour in little children are legion. One of its commonest expressions is in phobias and night terrors. When the little child wakens up, sweating and screaming with anxiety in the night, and says, " An animal bite my feet," we know that he is projecting on to the revived image of some real animal both his own biting aggression against his mother, feelings which cause him such profound distress and terror, and the " bad " biting vengeful mother of fantasy within him.   He says to her in effect, " It is not I who wish to bite you, it is Goo-goo who wants to bite me and you."   In this way he wins sympathy and protection from his mother, instead of the feared vengeance, and internal ease from the distress of knowing how strong his own biting urges are.   Such night-time fears, or some form of daytime phobias, are wellnigh universal from the second to the fourth years, although they vary greatly in intensity and frequency from one child to another.   They are one of the child's normal modes of maintaining internal psychic equilibrium in these years.

Every now and then one comes across a child who can express the nature of primitive fear so clearly that we are helped in our understanding of these deep-lying mental processes.   The mother of a little girl gave me the following instance recently.   At the age of twenty months the child saw a shoe of her mother's from which the sole had come loose and was flapping about.   The mother thought this would amuse the child.   But she was horrified, and for about a week would shrink away or shriek with terror if her mother wore shoes at all.   Eventually the mother bought a pair of brightly coloured house-shoes, and with much coaxing persuaded the child to unpack them and put them on her mother's feet.   For the next week or so the mother dared not wear any other shoes, and did not wear the particular offending pair again for several months. The child gradually forgot about it, but about fifteen months later she suddenly said in a frightened voice, " Where are Mummy's broken shoes ? " and then when her mother said hastily that she had sent them away, the child said, " They might have eaten me right up." One can readily understand how the flapping sole, with perhaps some nails sticking out, might appear like an open mouth with teeth, to a child of twenty months. But the actual resemblance is so slight and remote that one can only understand the intensity of the fear, and the fact that the child behaves as if the shoe really was a mouth that " might eat her up ", if one realizes that she is projecting her own biting impulses on to her mother's shoe. This fear of an external object is unpleasant enough to experience, but it has its compensations ; the frightening shoe can be removed and hidden away, in a way that one's own impulses cannot be, and the child can get effective help and protection from her mother and prove once again her love and sympathy, in a way that she feels would be impossible if her own aggressive wishes were known.

Another frequent piece of behaviour in which the process of projection plays a large part is the outbreak of obstinacy and temper tantrums. In these moments the child is again struggling with a fear of *internal* origin, but here it is not so much his own infantile wishes, which he now projects outwards, as the " bad ", primitively fantasied mother who will bite and rage against him from the inside. He is seeing that dangerous destructive internal mother in the person of the real mother or nurse, whom he defies in order to gain the real proof of security. Even if she, the real mother or nurse, is angry with him, even if she whips him, she does not actually tear him to pieces in the way he fears the " bad " mother within him will do, as he has wanted to do to her in the rages of infancy. And so he is supported against his worst terrors. These outbursts of temper and obstinacy are often very difficult to deal with. To the sensible and affectionate mother it seems inexplicable that the child should be so recalcitrant, so completely unreasonable, so untouched by persuasion or argument or even by punishment. But the child is not in fact struggling against the reasonable and sensible mother, not even against the mother who loses her temper and speaks sharply or smacks him. He is struggling against a far more primitive and absolute parent inside him, she who, he fears, will really damage him irreparably by biting and tearing. With a child who is well handled, these violent tantrums become more rare and less violent and unmanageable as he grows towards his fourth or fifth year. And this comes about just because he gets constant proof that his real parents have not the qualities of the fantasied internal mother, built in the image of the child himself. His mother's love and guidance in real skill gradually temper the terror of this raging infant-mother within him. And the child learns presently to adopt other more satisfactory modes of dealing with his internal problem of love and hate. Nevertheless, it is helpful to remember that even in these most difficult moments of rigid obstinacy and violent screaming, the child is not wholly given up to the destructive forces in himself. He is not in fact such an enemy to our educational purposes as it would seem on the surface. This is one of the major steps forward in his development, in spite of the fact that at first sight it may appear so retrogressive. It becomes genuinely retrogressive only if we handle the child badly. We encourage him to fly to this as a fixed mode of avoiding the intensest pain and terror if we are unreasonable or cruel in our dealing with him. The child may then have recourse to an excessive hate and defiance against the internal pain of remorse and guilt. In a lecture on " Rebellious Children " given about a year ago, I pointed out that, in dealing with delinquent children or with people whose characters have become set along lines of hate and defiance, we constantly find a special sensitivity to those issues of love and hate, hidden behind their outer shell of apparent hardness and lack of remorse. It is true that in such people the tendency to hate when frustrated appears to have been unusually strong from the beginning ; but it is not true that they lacked all feelings of love, and felt only hate. We invariably find that there was also strong and intense love ; but that the child could not bear the conflict between these two feelings. He could not tolerate the bitter grief and remorse of knowing that he hated and wanted to destroy the very person whom he also loved, and needed to cherish. When, in the work of analysis, we gently uncover, step by step, the old deep situations of difficulty, the need for excessive hate and defiance always disappears or

187

SUSAN ISAACS

greatly lessens.   The true lover may lie hidden even in the criminal.

It is his despair about controlling his aggressive feelings which drives the child to identify himself with the bad things, to say that these shall be triumphant.   From time to time every little child has this feeling ; but it only becomes a settled attitude in those children from whom the environment withholds love and understanding.   It would not become a characteristic way of life unless the child underwent really bad experiences—for example, the complete failure of adults to understand and help the child, or else their unkindness or cruelty, or some tragic loss.

The concrete fantasies underlying this attitude of mind are many and varied.   These can only be understood if we remember that in his earliest experiences, love *is* the good breast, the good milk, the good mother herself.   Both good and evil to the child are real, concrete things or persons.   Sometimes, for example, the child feels that love must be denied and covered up by hate and defiance, because there is not enough of it.   It is too little and too weak, and will only be wasted if one tries to use it. The only hope of preserving love may be to keep it hidden away inside one, never to draw upon one's resources.   In the future perhaps one may bring it out and use it ; but not now.   If one used it now, there would be nothing left for the future.   Again, the child may feel that it is better to bring out all the bad *first*, to make sure, for example, that his mother knows how bad he is before he trusts her to love him.   If she seems to love him because she

188

thinks he is altogether good, then, presently, she may discover how much bàd he also has in him, and then will cease to love him. Or if he does not bring all the bad out (for example, his fæces and urine) before he tries to get her good things into him (her love and her milk), then his bad will destroy all her good. The feeling that the bad and the good must never be mixed up is extremely strong in some children, and accounts for much open naughtiness. Quite simple and concrete unconscious notions such as this are always to be found underlying excessive hatred and defiance in the behaviour of the little child or the character of the grown-up.

In his struggle with his own impulses of love and hate, his own bodily substances, and his immense need to control these as well as to make his real parents minister to his life and need of love, the child comes to feel that he must be stronger than these forces, external and internal. You all know how little children love to climb up on top of things, for example, a wall or chest of drawers, and say, " Now I'm bigger than you," how the tiny child delights in being able to make his father or mother do what he wants, for example, to go on picking up the toy he throws down, or pretend to be weak and helpless while he drives them before him ; or how he loves to stand in dramatic attitudes and pretend he is the policeman controlling the traffic, or the driver managing the bus. In all these ways, we see the need of the little child to be stronger than the people and objects in his world, whether the real ones outside him or the fantasied ones inside.

Every child shows this from time to time in an endless variety of ways, and it is a very important element in dramatic play. This omnipotent attitude is one of the ways out of the despair which the child feels when he cannot control or get rid of his aggressive impulses towards his good mother. In effect, he says, " I *must* be ' on top of things ', *must* be able to control them." Such an attitude is all very well when worked out in playful drama ; but if it becomes a settled way of life, it often means that the child is unable to learn or to accept the help he so much needs. In order to learn and to accept help one has to be humble, to be able to admit one's own ignorance and lack of skill. One has to believe in the possibility of *learning* to control, and not to imagine or assert that one is already in control, when the facts belie this feeling. The child who *must* feel himself cleverer or bigger than his father will obviously not be able to learn much from him. Such an attitude is a common ingredient in backwardness in learning at school, as well as in social aloofness and unfriendliness. You will readily see that carping and criticism, or any emphasis upon the child's ignorance, does not help him to overcome this special difficulty. Confident encouragement and an understanding of any special points of difficulty or confusion, making steps easy for him and showing him that it is possible to be a learner and yet to be respected, will often, however, help him out of this impasse.

This brings us to another general movement of the child's mind, of the utmost possible importance for his growth and education, one whose outer aspects are perfectly familiar to us in the child's wish to learn and to achieve, but whose deeper roots we have only come to understand through the work of psycho-analysis. This is the (unconscious) wish to restore and make restitution to the mother, who has, in real or fantasied behaviour, been damaged or hurt (for example, by biting, wetting or dirtying). This is a powerful motive in the forward movement of the child's growth, underlying every aspect of his development in skill and knowledge and affection and social ease. In his deepest fantasy, it is the wish to give back to the breast the milk which has been taken from it, to give his mother children and health and youth, to bring her and his father together in happy and fruitful intercourse. And the child wishes to restore not only the real external mother, but the mother in himself, as the source of all good in him. On this earliest level, to restore the mother *is* to restore himself, and indeed to restore the whole world, since in the earliest days, self and world are one. Every time the little child tries to put one block on another, to wash his own hands, to speak and sing, he is expressing (among other wishes and purposes) this desire to make whole the mother within him, to deny or restore the results of his biting, dirtying or screaming.

One of the biggest sources of trouble for the little child is precisely that at the time when his need to make things better is the most intense and urgent, his skill in doing this is so much less than the ease with which he can destroy. At eighteen months and two years it is so easy to dirty, to knock things down, to make a mess with one's food, to scream

and shout. It is so difficult, indeed almost impossible, to make things clean, to build and draw, even
to speak or sing in a way that brings pleasure to
oneself or others. Many children are overcome by
the sense of the insufficiency of the good within
them to counterbalance the bad; and this despair
very largely rests on this real lack of skill and knowledge. This, again, is why children so often have
to play at being bigger and wiser and cleverer than
they are. They have to be on top of things in imagination because they do not know how to achieve
in reality. Provided their faith is kept alive, however, this contrast lessens step by step. One of the
biggest changes that occurs in the child between
one and four years of age is the growth in confidence
in his own skill and in the possibility of real achievement, whether in making things or speaking or giving pleasure to others. Everything we can do to
further the child's development of bodily skill, of
artistic expression, of confidence in his power to
help others and gain pleasure from their company,
will aid his struggle with the destructive forces inside
himself, and carry him out of the despair that confirms him in his destructiveness and defiance. Tantrums and obstinacies and night terrors thus gradually get less, not so much by the direct comfort we
give to the child at the time, as by the indirect support against the very source of these things, which
he gains by his normal growth in the arts of life.
Much could be said about the immense psychological
value of the little child's play, and of all his impulses
to learn and to do. Many of you are already familiar
with the remarkable changes in health and peace of

mind which a good nursery school will effect for the child of three or four years. It does this by means of providing the right materials and the right opportunities for the child's own normal impulses to skill and achievement, thus giving him a profound reassurance against his inner doubts and difficulties and depressions.

We cannot understand these difficulties unless we appreciate the remorselessness of a little child's logic, and the way in which his ignorance of physical causes and events in the real world confirms his worst fears of the power of his own bad wishes. When two things happen together in the experience of a little child, they are felt by him to be causally related. If, for example, his mother is ill or the new baby should die just after he has had an outburst of temper (or even after he has felt a spasm of hatred against his mother or the baby), then the illness or death is for his mind the direct outcome of his own behaviour or his own secret wishes. In the analysis of every adult, whether normal or neurotic, one finds endless examples of this infantile logic. If tragic events occur, it may become so remorseless and inescapable that the child's life is dominated by the feeling that the only way of restoring the life of the baby brother would be to die himself. I have known some extraordinarily clear instances of this, in which the whole course of the later life of the individual was determined by a mental process of this kind. Whether one calls it a fantasy or a primitive logical process is immaterial : what is important is that all the rest of life may be organized around the denial or postponement of what is felt to be an inevitable event, one's own death, as the only means of restoring the loved mother or her child. A striking instance of this kind was told to me recently by a head mistress of an infant school. A group of children sometimes played at being Red Indians. One child was chosen as the victim of an attack, and was to be killed, cut up and eaten. The head mistress noticed with what complete passivity a particular boy always gave himself up to the rôle of victim. Indeed, it was more than passivity. He entered into it with such complete abandonment that she was quite troubled by his attitude. It was as if he existed to be sacrificed in this way, and whenever the play, or one of a similar kind, was repeated, he contrived to be the chosen victim, always wearing an air of deep satisfaction throughout. Inquiries brought out a significant piece of early history. When this boy was about two and a half he actually saw his little brother of about a year younger fall from an upper window of the house and be killed. It became clear that in this play which had arrested the attention of the head mistress, the boy was fulfilling a demand of his own inner life that he should die in his turn and thus expiate the death of the younger brother. A few days later, he told another mistress that when he was grown up he was " going to be a boxer so as to get killed ". The boy's inner life was evidently dominated by the terrible sight he had seen as a small child, and by his feeling that this event had come about as the result of his own wishes against the rival brother.

One observes the same situation even more clearly in the actual analysis of some small children in whose life there have been distressing real events. The boy of four, for example, whom I quoted in the previous chapter, revealed the most intense wish to die as the only basis on which things could be made better again for those whom he loved. This appeared in the analysis after a series of very unfortunate happenings in the boy's home. Within the space of one week, a week which happened to be the anniversary of his father's death, his aunt seriously injured an arm, his mother badly scalded her foot, and his grandmother had to go into a hospital for an operation for cataract. At the end of this period his mother caught a bad cold, and brought the child to the Clinic in response to my having pointed out his urgent need for psychological help, on a day when she herself was not fit to be about. The boy was terribly distressed by the fact that all these bad things had happened in his home, and connected them not only with his own destructive wishes, but with the analysis and myself. The fact that I wanted his mother to bring him to the Clinic even when she herself had a cold turned me into a bad and dangerous person. How could I make him better if I was so cruel as to make his mother come out when she was ill ? This identified me with the "bad" Daddy who did not come alive in order to help her, who by his death made her have to work hard to earn money for the boy and was not able to help her or him in any way. If I was so bad to the mother I could not possibly be good to him, and he showed by his behaviour that he was in very great terror of me as a person who was (in his fantasy) responsible for all these bad happenings. He had already shown me that he felt he ought to be shot at, drowned, exposed so as to die, instead of his father, and thus bring the latter alive to help his mother, since he could not himself help her. On this particular day when his mother came with the cold, he reproached me openly for not making her better. When I greeted him with a smile, he said bitterly, " *Why* do you laugh ? " He broke every toy that could in any way represent his father or himself, he stood in a corner and, with complete detachment from me and the external world, reproached the fantasied father inside him, saying in a bitter voice, " Yes, you *are* a cruel Daddy." He then took a bowl of water and attempted to pour it down inside his jersey on to his own chest, in order to give himself (or rather the " bad Daddy " inside him) the cold that his mother was suffering from. When I prevented this action, he turned the water over me, since by preventing him from attacking the bad Daddy and so saving his mother, I myself became identified with that bad father.

These instances are specially dramatic ones, and I quote them because of their content, and because they demonstrate how complex and intense are the thoughts and feelings of even a very young child about what happens to himself and those whom he loves. Fortunately not every child experiences such tragic happenings. The real experiences of most children fortify them against their worst fantasies and lead them to realize that they can help to make things better. Nevertheless, the essential problem

is there for every child. Such bad happenings as
do occur are related by the child to his aggressive
impulses, and taken as confirmations of his worst
fears. The way in which we ourselves deal with
problems of operations and illnesses and deaths in
speaking to the child will thus obviously make a
very great difference to him.

At an earlier point I spoke of the little child's
intense feelings of rivalry to other children, but I
pointed out also that the arrival of a new baby is
not a source of fear and depression only. These
feelings of fear and depression may be the first
reaction, but after a time at any rate, the little
brother or sister becomes a great source of comfort
against the child's worst fantasies. And in his play
and companionship with other children lies one of
the most powerful means of social and emotional
education for the young child. The value of such
companionship is to be understood not only in terms
of conscious experience and the deliberate education
we give to the child by means of it, but also through
its unconscious significance. You will remember
that all these fantasies and movements of the child's
mind which I am describing are mostly unconscious.
Nevertheless, they are most intimately affected by
real events and real experiences. There is indeed
a continuous interplay between unconscious fantasy
and real experience. The ways in which his play
with his fellows helps the child both consciously
and unconsciously are manifold and it would be
too long a story to describe them here.

Observations of the child's behaviour in the
nursery school confirm all that we have discovered

about his inner life from the process of individual analysis. It has often been noticed how the two-year-old, for example, who enters a group of other children, either at a friend's home or in the nursery school, will cling to an adult and watch the other children with round observant eyes without attempting to join in their activities. This watchful suspicion is presently followed by a period of rather boisterous and aggressive contact in which he pushes and pulls and perhaps pinches or smacks the other children, clearly with an air of discovering what may happen. This active hostility is the first step on the path towards sharing the play of other children and learning to be really friendly and co-operative. In the first phase, other children are simply felt to be rivals and enemies. All one's own aggression is projected on to them, and one remains entirely defensive and watching, with the support of a helpful grown-up. The second phase is an active testing of one's own and other people's behaviour, in order to see what does happen as a result of real participation. But since one has not yet learnt to be social and co-operative, all one can do at first is to push and pull. Laughter and friend-liness often accompany these apparently aggressive acts, however, and it is by means of these same aggressive interchanges with other children that the child learns that others are not wholly hostile. They do not eat him up, but can be played with safely. And then comes the active pleasure and real support of playing with them.

When a child recognizes the possibility of identifying himself with others of his own age and skill, he feels that he has a new support against those adults of whom he is a little afraid, in the real world, or the frightening " bad " parent inside his own mind. Once they have discovered the pleasure of togetherness, children will do all sorts of things together that they never dared do alone. By means of this alliance, they gain support against the grown-ups, who are overwhelming not only because they may be angry and punishing, but also by virtue of their good qualities and the child's complete dependence upon them. The child now tastes the pleasure of social contacts, of physical helpfulness as well as talk and play, and so the world gradually becomes peopled with at least as many friends as enemies, and with an increasing number of sources of active delight. The fact that children can give each other pleasure of one form or another is a very important aid to their development, both as an end in itself and as a support against fears of only being able to dirty and damage. If other children bestow admiration one cannot after all be wholly weak and inferior. The help which the companionship of other children thus brings can, however, only be realized if the child's experience with them is real and active. Their mere presence without active contact will not do this for him. If the adult rules with a rod of iron and determines all the contacts of children with each other, if he will not allow them to develop mutual loyalties, if he pounces at once on the slightest sign of anger or quarrelsomeness, if he interferes too much with their naïve expressions of play and love, then the existence of other children will not do much for anyone.

In this connection we are often asked about the sexual play of little children, whether they should be allowed to admire each other's naked bodies or look at or touch each other's genitals, or to play those favourite lavatory games of " doctor " and " mother and baby ".

This is a very difficult question to answer and no simple and general rule can be laid down about it. Sexual gratification of some sort is a normal element in a healthy mental life at every age. Games of the kinds mentioned are extremely common in the early years, so much so that they are commonly overlooked. With children over five, they tend to be less common, but even then are much more frequent than most people realize. Such sexual play may be a means, and sometimes (for internal reasons) the only means, the child has of establishing pleasurable contacts with his peers and comforting himself against his own fears of badness, and thus laying the foundation of future happiness in adult sexual life. When these things happen between children of about the same age and are entered upon willingly by each partner, there is no reason to think that they do any harm, and most often they undoubtedly do great good. Nevertheless, they may give rise to difficulty with particular children, by stirring up too great guilt or anxiety, owing to their special and individual meaning. Above all, sexual experience may be harmful if it is forced upon one child by another, or if the companions are of different ages. A seduction forced upon a younger child by an older can sometimes have almost as serious a psychological effect as if the seducer were an adult. It is therefore by no means easy to offer general advice, although it is certain that harsh interference with the child's play and curiosities may make him afraid of all physical forms of love, unable to fulfil his normal sexual functions in later life, and uneasy in his social contacts. It may confirm his worst fears about the badness of his own and other people's bodies, and of sexual impulses generally.

On the other hand, there is no doubt that it would not help the child to *encourage* his sexual plays, since it is always difficult to know just what these mean to him. Certainly we should avoid creating, out of our own ignorance or unwillingness to recognize the sexuality of children, such situations as will expose them to severe temptation of a kind that would be on the whole more harmful than not —for example, by allowing an adolescent boy and a little girl to share the same room.

When the child, moreover, shows his sexual activities openly before adults (at any rate after the first four or five years), this nearly always means that sexual play is being used to cover up a very acute anxiety. An older child who masturbates openly or exposes his genital, or talks about sexual matters in front of the grown-ups apparently without any reserve or shame, is usually asking for help against his difficulties. This is a different situation from the naïve pleasure of younger children in each others' bodies, which after three or four years of age they normally tend to hide away from adults.

Perhaps the best general rule is to turn a blind eye to the talk and play of little children in these directions, leaving it to them to work out their problems for themselves, save where the sexual element becomes so blatant and defiant and directed to the grown-ups that it seems clear that the child is deliberately drawing attention to it because he wants it to be stopped, or wants to be helped against his fears of it. As Mrs. Klein suggested in her footnote on page 47, an attitude of easy tolerance of the child's sexuality, without encouraging it or entering into it, is the best help that the adult can give in the ordinary way.

In general, then, learning to play, to talk, to fantasy, to work, together with other children is an essential means of emotional balance and growth in little children of the nursery years.

In all his varied contacts with other children and with grown-up friends and relatives, which the child enjoys in the normal home, he discovers another aid to his internal life. All his feelings are, as we have seen, focused at first upon his mother, and then upon his nurse and father. But these other social experiences lead to a gradual diffusion of his emotions, which thus become less intense and less unmanageable. These varied contacts with aunts and uncles and visitors and playmates give the child the opportunity to compare and test not only one person with another, but the outer realities with the inner images. And so his feelings and impulses are gradually brought under the control of knowledge and experience, and gain a perspective and proportion that the child could not easily attain if his real experience was confined to his own parents.

Let me now briefly review these major tendencies in the child's mind which I have instanced, enabling him gradually to master his first great welter of intense feelings, and by turning a part of his emotions, now in this direction, now in that, to lessen the central conflict and thus slowly stabilize his inner life.

I described, first, the way in which he separates the " good " and the " bad " aspects of his own feelings and of his primitively conceived mother, and projects and displaces these, now the one and now the other, on to the various real persons of his outer world. By means of this diffusion, the tension of feelings is lessened, and he is enabled to see more clearly and to act more adaptively. This " splitting " and displacement of feeling do not, however, lead automatically to further development. Their work needs to be carried forward by those other psychological agencies which I have described. If the child's real experience is bad in the earliest years, then it may happen that he will learn to keep the " good " hidden away within him and to turn all his own " bad " outwards. He will then all the more need to find people who can be (or seem) to him absolutely good, to protect him against the dangers of the absolutely " bad ", the fairy godmother or prince who will save him from the witches and ogres. But he will never for long be able to trust in these fantastically " good " helpers. They will only too soon lose their safety for him and become in their turn objects of suspicion and distrust. If, on the other hand, the real people in his early environment are even-tempered and controlled, able to take care of themselves and manage his aggression, whilst yet remaining loving and understanding and fostering his skills, he will gradually lose his fear of his own impulses and his own fantasies.

His contacts with other friendly grown-ups, father, nurse and relatives, will lead him out of the closed circle of his first ambivalence towards his mother, diffusing and articulating his feelings by linking them with a variety of real experiences.

I described at some length the vast unconscious significance of the child's wish to acquire real skills, the discovery that he can express his deepest impulses in forms that give pleasure to other people, in creative art, in rhythm and song and speech, and that he can learn to make and do, and not only to repair real or fantasied damage, but actually to create new objects. I showed how the birth of brothers and sisters or the companionship of other children in the nursery school carries further these various lines of development, and gradually leads the child into the world of real social achievements and satisfactions.

These are some of the more important unconscious processes which underlie the great change in the external aspects of the child's behaviour as he passes through the years of the nursery. Gradually, and with many temporary crises of difficulty, he changes from the self-centred infant bound in the circle of his own wishes and fears and fantasies, limited in every direction by lack of strength and skill and knowledge, to the independent but socialized child of six or seven who is able to assert himself against grown-ups or other children and yet to remain loving and friendly ; who has left behind most of his phobias and obstinacies, and knows that he can learn and make and do in the real world. The degree to which his development is satisfactory will very largely depend upon the extent to which the environment has furthered these forward-moving tendencies in his mind, or hampered and forced him back towards the more primitive infantile modes of response.

I must now turn to practical considerations, and consider very briefly such suggestions as psycho-analysis can offer regarding the best ways of making the nursery a true community, a place where the child is helped forward not only to social life, but to internal security and harmony also.

Already in passing I have made a number of fragmentary comments on practical issues. I want now to gather these together, and to summarize them more systematically. In the main I have so far emphasized the fantasy life of the child, the psychic processes through which his experiences gain their meanings for him. Now, however, I must emphasize more directly the external reality, the real differences in the behaviour of one person and another, one circumstance and another, and the effect these have upon the child's power to deal with his internal problems.

In the first place, all that I have said will have emphasized the value and importance of realizing how extraordinarily *human* babies and little children are. If only we could give little children the same degree of consideration as we naturally extend to adults, we should be able to avoid many of our worst mistakes. I am not suggesting that we should treat the infant and young child as if they were adults. They are not. Their needs are in many essential ways very different ; but if we avoid making the extraordinary assumption that they are mere reflex machines and have no feelings or mental needs, we shall then be willing to take pains to understand what those feelings and needs are. Babies are immature human beings, but human all the same. External events mean more to them, not less. Our voices and manners and personalities affect children more intensely and immediately than they do our grown-up friends and relatives. Yet whilst we are willing to take endless trouble to make a guest feel at home, to avoid hurting the feelings of a grown-up member of the family, or to extend the right expressions of sympathy to someone who has suffered a tragic loss, we are too often ready to let children endure all these things without the slightest understanding or help from us. For example, to suit our own purposes, we light-heartedly dismiss a nurse to whom the child has become attached. Or if a devoted nurse has to leave for good reasons, we do not try to imagine what an overwhelming loss this must be for the child. We demand expressions of politeness from him that we never offer to him. We expect him to love us and to love us best, as a matter of course, without doing anything to win his affection, as we certainly should do with an adult whom we wished to win. We ask him annoying questions when he is not in the mood to answer them—in a way we should think incredibly rude to an adult. We talk about him in front of him, and sometimes even relate our own triumphs over him in a way which would lead us to be ostracized in adult society. We quarrel in front of him, as if it meant nothing to him to have the most important grown-ups in his environment hurting each other. We do this and at the same time expect him to be considerate and polite and loving to us and to other children. Fortunately, not every parent makes all these mistakes. You know that in bringing all these errors together in one picture, I am offering a caricature of the ordinary sensible and affectionate parent. But most of us make some of these mistakes, and the ordinary sensible and affectionate parent is liable to fall into them just when they matter most. There seems to be something deep within the minds of us adults which leads us persistently to under-estimate the reality of the child's feelings, to assume that he cannot hear and see, or is not listening, or not concerned with what we do and say and are. Yet it is precisely these general attitudes, these pervading modes of behaviour towards the child that affect his feelings towards us, far more than our explicit statements of our didactic purposes towards him. It is in these ways that we show what we really are in ourselves. I do not believe that we can begin to help the little child unless we remember that all those major events such as partings and losses and loves and deaths, on the one hand, and all those involuntary and constant expressions of our own attitudes towards him on the other, affect him profoundly in his deepest feelings. They do so all the more because, whilst human, he is immature.

The child does see and hear and feel, and he does

remember. In analytic work with adults, one is never able to get altogether used to the extraordinary tenacity of memory and profundity of feeling which is retained throughout life with regard to the earliest events, at one or two or three years of age. These are perhaps hidden under an apparent blank, or distorted out of recognition, but they are always there, and always have a profound and permanent effect upon later development. It is incredible to the psycho-analyst that anyone can take the view that what happens at one or two years of age does not matter. A mother recently told me of how she had gone to a well-known institution for training nurses, to ask if they could supply a nurse who had some psychological understanding of infants, as well as being expert in physical care. The matron's reply was, " Psychology *for a nurse of a baby of one year*? What ridiculous nonsense! "

It was reported in the papers not so very long ago how the parents of a baby of fifteen months who had had a terrible experience prosecuted the owner of the animal which had caused the infant this suffering. A large monkey had escaped from a private zoo and had jumped on to the child sleeping in his perambulator in the garden and tormented him. When the case was tried for damages, a doctor was brought forward by the defendant, who said that such an event would not have the slightest effect upon the infant's mind, since at fifteen months he was far too young to remember these things ! Nothing could be further from the truth. Unless expert psychological help were available, it is safe to predict that this experience would have a serious and a deleterious effect upon the emotional development of the child in later life. Little that did not involve actual physical injury could be of more serious psychological purport than this event for a child of one year. It is an extremely interesting and profound psychological problem in itself, to ask what are the psychological forces in us, which lead us to blot out so completely from our common psychic experience all this vast area of the first two or three years of life.

The second point I want to make is the great value to the little child of a firm background of regular routine and quiet control. Nowadays we are familiar with the gain to the child's physical health of a regular life, but we do not always realize what this means to him psychologically. A well-ordered rhythm in the day's routine gives the infant a general feeling of emotional security. Many children show great distress if the usual series of events is disturbed in any way, for example, by a change of hour for the meal or the bath, a different order in dressing or feeding him. Some, indeed, show such an acute intolerance of change that one feels this is already a neurotic symptom. But there are few who do not thrive better when their life is well and regularly planned.

The child's love of rhythm and pattern in the general course of the day is but one instance of his search for rhythm and pattern in his life as a whole. We have all noticed how little children delight in rhythmic movements, in sucking and rocking, rhythmic crooning, the old lullabies and repetitive nursery rhymes, swinging and dancing. These bring a profound harmony and peace to the child, by imposing order upon the chaos of feeling as well as upon bodily movements. In the child's unconscious fantasy, rhythm brings together into a whole things that are otherwise scattered, disordered, broken bits. The rhythmic sounds of speech or of song, for instance, create beauty and evoke love, whereas noises and screams shatter the air and the ear, and stir up fear and hatred. There is a profound wisdom in the child's feeling that rhythm is life.

The order which he needs is, however, not only one of meals and rest times, coming and going by the clock. Even more deeply and urgently, he seeks a stable pattern in his relations with people. He can be secure and content only if there is a harmony of feeling amongst those who make up his world, towards him and towards each other. If the grown-ups are changeable towards him, loving one moment, teasing the next, angry one day and indulgent another, the infant feels bewildered and lost. If they break promises to him, if they demand immediate obedience in one breath and then with the next give way and become complacent when he storms and defies them, if they adopt one method to-day and another the next, the child is left without guide or anchor. He cannot predict what sort of feeling and behaviour his own actions will evoke in them; and since he has nothing to go upon but his actual experience in learning to order his own feelings and impulses, how can he then have faith in the possibility of order within himself? When grown-ups are haphazard and incalculable, the child feels that *he* has made everything messy and broken everything to pieces. His lack of trust in his own power to create and control is strengthened, and his belief in the destructive power of his wishes and his bodily substances is confirmed.

Not seldom mothers of difficult children say in desperation, " I have tried every method I have heard of. I have scolded him and bribed him and coaxed him and punished him, and I have tried taking no notice, and nothing I do seems to have the slightest effect." They do not realize that such *changes* of attitude are themselves extremely puzzling and frightening to the little child. He cannot know why he is scolded one day and coaxed the next and ignored on the third. What he *experiences* is that his mother is not to be depended upon. She gives him no sense of rhythm or order or security. I sometimes feel that almost any reasonably humane method would be more successful for the child if it were followed out in an orderly and systematic way than frequent choppings and changes in ill-considered attempts to discover the best method. The child is just as aware as the mother herself of her desperate sense that she does not know how to treat him, and he becomes convinced that she has no help to give him.[1]

[1] We must of course not overlook the equally great dangers of a fixed unbending attitude and over-rigid rules. If we hold firmly to a settled and considered general mode of treating the child and if our general attitude towards him is stable, we may then leave ourselves free to adapt ourselves to his special needs from day to day and to make any detailed changes in our methods of treating him that the situation seems to call for. A stable love and understanding will allow plenty of room for minor variations as the child's own emotional needs fluctuate.

This is the deepest and most significant ground for sustaining an ordered pattern in the physical care of the child and in our own ways of feeling and behaving towards him, namely, that these things strengthen his belief in the goodness of his own life and his own ability to love and create.

They have, however, other meanings too. An orderly background and the quiet control of the child's life by his parents means to him that they accept at any rate some of the responsibility for controlling his destructive wishes, and they do this without fulfilling his awful fantasies of the vengeful " bad " parents within him. They enable him to project upon external reality his inner fantasies of the " bad " mother and thus to measure and test these fantasies by reality, gaining the assurance that it is possible to be checked and controlled without being hurt. You all know how certain children will seek actively to provoke resistance and denial or punishment from their parents by open and persistent defiance. When an expression of disapproval has been won, such children seem to feel for a time more secure, since they have once again proved that real parents do not necessarily destroy when they are angry. The more difficult children have to keep on behaving in such a way as to get these reassurances constantly, although the feeling of comfort does not last very long. The more ordinary child can find the reassurance he needs in the milder control of a regular life and the quiet but firm limit which every sensible parent will set upon the real aggression and the real expression of destructive impulses.

The child, moreover, seeks to prove not merely that his parents will not eat him up or destroy him, but also that they will not let him eat them up or injure them irremediably. When the more difficult child persists in his naughtiness until he is checked or punished, a very strong motive in his behaviour is his wish to receive certain proof that his parents will set a limit *for their own sakes* ; in other words, that they will and can defend themselves against his destructive impulses towards them.

These three meanings which mild and gentle control may have for the child will be blended in very varying emphasis in different children. Together they form the chief psychological basis for the contentment shown by the little child whose parents are firm and sure in their control of him, as well as able to maintain a rhythmic harmony in his external forms of living.

We must, however, at once add another point, one which requires even greater emphasis than the last since it is far more commonly neglected or un-understood, namely, that such control, if it is to help the child, needs to be based upon an adequate understanding of the child's own impulses of growth. Its aim should not be the negative one, for example, of mere obedience, but the positive one of enabling the child to develop his own real gifts and achievements. If we treat the child as dis-obedient because he wants to learn to feed himself, if we check his desire to become skilful and in-dependent in washing his own hands or in express-ing his own view of the world in drawing and modelling, for fear of the mess he may make in the doing, if we value more highly a quiet demeanour at the meal table than free and friendly talk about his interests, if in general we prefer the forms of external order to the signs of genuine growth in skill and understanding, then our control of the child will act adversely, no matter how mild the sanctions with which we exercise it. It is of immense aid to the child when the mother recognizes his need to learn and to do, and provides the right materials and opportunities for his activity. In his efforts to run and climb and jump and dance, to model and paint, to sing and speak, to read and write, the child is not merely seeking external skills or imitating grown-up people in an external way. He is, more than anything else, seeking to keep the " good " parents alive within himself by becoming as helpful and as understanding as they are. All those most profound forces of the deepest levels of the child's mind, which I have attempted to describe, are at work in his wish to learn and grow. Earlier in this chapter, I referred to those little children who are so afraid of making messes and spoiling things, so distressed because they cannot do things as perfectly as their parents, that they can only pretend to do things, and will not even try to learn and do in reality. Such children can see only two possibilities, being helpless and destructive children, or powerful and entirely perfect parents. If they cannot at once become the latter by an act of magical incorporation, they yield themselves up to the despair of being for ever destructive, messy children. All they can achieve in the way of saving the world from the effects of their badness is to keep perfectly still and learn and do nothing. Now if we ourselves set standards that are too high for the child, judge his first efforts too severely, see the fault instead of the effort, we strengthen these unreal attitudes in him. The child certainly values a just judgment from us; he does not want us to say things are well if they are ill, or to indulge him against our own better judgment. But he needs to feel that we can look under and through his errors to the love and genuine effort that may lie behind them. Every detail of the way in which we try to teach him such things as manners and polite conversation, independence in tending himself or school attainments, will affect his own trust in us and in his growing powers.

It has been my experience that mere lack of knowledge on the part of many parents of what is to be expected of the ordinary child at any particular age is responsible for many serious faults in handling. Many mothers and nurses and fathers who are full of genuine goodwill towards their children make things harder for them by demanding standards of behaviour that are really unsuitable for the child's age. For example, many people expect even two-year-olds to sit still at table, or demand that a four-year-old child shall walk quietly beside his parents. But to sit still or to walk quietly and restrainedly is a very difficult task for a young child—much more so than for an older child or an adult. Little children run more readily and more naturally than they walk, and with far less strain on their co-ordinating mechanisms. And they learn to talk well far more easily than they learn to be silent. We starve their belief in us and in themselves when we demand things that not only lead to immediate failure but close the normal avenues of love and achievement. It is thus of the greatest value to parents to gain a comparative knowledge of the norms of achievement in all the ordinary personal skills and language, since this alone will bring a just perspective of the behaviour of their own children.

And this applies not only to skills in a narrow sense, but to the broader issues of social adaptation as well. Many mothers, for instance, are worried because a child of two is shy of strangers ; because a child of four romances with long tales about things he has seen or things he desires which bear no relation to the facts ; because a child of six and a half is inclined to be stubborn and to turn a deaf ear to the things the adults want of him ; or again, because a boy of fifteen or sixteen begins to assert his own opinion dogmatically over against his father's views. In each case they fail to realize the normality of this behaviour at the given age and its value as an index of a forward mental movement. In any case, it is better to err in the direction of leniency and expecting too little than in the direction of demands that are beyond the child's capacity.

One particular problem about which such ignorance is widespread and causes perhaps the greatest difficulty is that of masturbation. Those who are engaged in advisory work are constantly approached by mothers and nurses who are disturbed because a boy or girl, of any age beyond the first year, is masturbating in some way or another. Parents regard this as an unusual and very abnormal occurrence, and recount the various attempts they have made to stop it. Very rarely indeed have they any knowledge of the fact that masturbation is, in some form or another, practically universal in children. It is an enormous help to mothers and nurses when they realize that this is not a secret and abnormal occurrence with their own particular children, but a normal and harmless happening with children generally, although it varies in the age of incidence and in intensity. Merely to know this sets it in a better perspective, since what mothers and nurses fear is that it will do harm, and that the children will, because of this, grow up to be generally abnormal.

From all that has been said in this and earlier chapters, it will be clear to readers that masturbation is an expression of complex mental processes in the child. In the first place, it is a simple expression of the child's own sexuality, an enjoyment normal to his age. Secondly, the pleasure he gains serves as a proof to the child that he has a " good " mother and father within him. To interfere directly with the relief and pleasure he gains in this way is always undesirable. In the majority of children the need to seek this special sort of comfort becomes much less urgent as they gain increasing enjoyment and reassurance in other ways (for example, various modes of play with external objects), and as their real social relations with other children expand and become more secure. In children who are suffering very considerable mental stress, masturbation tends to become compulsive and incessant Even

217

then the masturbation itself should not be interfered with, but the deeper causes of this excessive need for it discovered and remedied. Sometimes some change that gives the child a greater belief in himself, such as better opportunities to play, or more active signs of affection from parents, will relieve the unconscious tendencies which find expression in this way. The masturbating child thus calls for special help, not because he is doing harm to himself, but because he is showing us that he has some deep anxiety which can only be allayed in this manner.

This problem of masturbation is, as I have shown, but one of the examples which illustrate the value of a wide comparative knowledge of the behaviour of children at different ages and in varying circumstances. The general point I am attempting to make clear is that, whilst we need to give the little child the certainty that we will support him and defend ourselves against his destructive impulses, we need also to give him positive help towards his constructive wishes, the opportunity and material and understanding appropriate in detail at each age and phase of development. We cannot do this unless we are willing to acquaint ourselves with the facts of normal physical, intellectual and social growth.

I have spoken a good deal of providing for the child's learning. You will not, however, take me to refer only to school learning, or to the deliberate teaching of particular skills. The child's own spontaneous activities in his natural play are even more valuable to him. This is one of the directions in which the work of Melanie Klein has so greatly enlarged our psychological knowledge. Educators of genius have long recognized the immense value of the child's play for his general growth ; but it has been left for the deeper understanding of psycho-analysis to show fully what its precise psychological functions are.

Space will not allow me to amplify these here. I will content myself with mentioning three considera-tions. Firstly, in his play the child is able to elabo-rate his libidinal wishes and creative fantasies. Play gives him immense pleasure, and this alone would be its sufficient justification. Secondly, he gains enormous benefit from the opportunity to express his aggressive impulses and fantasies of punishment, without doing real harm. He can, for example, knock bricks down, squash a piece of plasticine, pretend to be a dangerous animal or a robber, run away from pursuing bears or giants, and can act all this out with vivid feeling and yet at the end of it know that he has hurt no real person, and thus has no reason to fear real retaliation. Thirdly, the child can, in his play, work out his restitutive impulses, his wish to make things better and restore all the harm his aggression has done, long before he is able to do this in reality. To play at being a good mother, a clever father, an efficient policeman or bus conductor, keeps alive in the child his belief in the " good " parents within him, and in fact gives him endless opportunities for real achievement by the way.

Whatever aspect of the child's life one is con-sidering, whether his external relations with people and things or his growth towards inner harmony, it is his own free dramatic play which brings him the greatest help. In the child's play are the seeds of all creative effort, of all art and science and philosophy; and in no way can we more fully show ourselves to the child as good and understanding parents than by helping him to find himself in his play.

You are familiar with the fact that it is by means of play that the child's analyst comes to understand and to relieve his difficulties in the analytic work. Even those psychotherapists, however, who do not work upon analytic lines (who do not, that is to say, put into words those deep and difficult things which the child struggles to express in his play), nevertheless find that inhibited or unhappy children benefit greatly from the mere opportunity to play in a friendly atmosphere, and with expressive material. Those children are in the greatest need of help who, for inner or outer reasons, cannot play at all.

The recognition of the psychological value of play leads us to another consideration. Very little children will often play alone. Still more often, however, they want others to play with them. Even the infant of a year or fifteen months searches eagerly for a grown-up companion in his play, and protests bitterly against being forced to lie alone or stay immobile in a pen. The child of two and three years wants other human beings around him even if he is occupying himself with solitary fantasy, and the child of three and four and onwards requires the companionship of other children almost as much as he needs physical care and the love of adults. This point brings us very close to the main consideration of this chapter as a whole : namely, the nursery as a community. Some companionship of other children in play is essential for a normal balance of the inner life and for successful outer adjustment. If the nursery is not a community in this sense it needs to be made so. If the child has no brothers and sisters of his own, he needs plenty of friends or a group of children who come at regular periods to share his activities. To illustrate one point, it has often been noticed how even acute difficulties about eating in an only child will disappear as soon as he takes his meals with other children in a group of friends or a nursery school. This will not be surprising to you if you remember what I said earlier about the various ways in which the child gains security against his fantastic terrors by living contact with his fellows.

In broadest outline, I have now given you what seem to me the main desiderata for healthy development. If we can provide these in their manifold detail of day-to-day experience, we are giving the child a maximum help towards overcoming his primary difficulties, and learning to trust in the active expression of his love and in active contact with other human beings.

Two further points must now be made. The first is that, as far as we possibly can, we should avoid allowing the child to be subjected to more than one source of emotional strain at any one time. I spoke at an earlier point of the way in which the primitive feeling-logic of the child leads him to feel that things happening together are causally connected. If we remember this, we shall be willing to go out of our way to prevent things happening to the child which might give rise to such feelings. For instance, it is not very wise to send a child away to a nursery school immediately after the birth of a younger child. From one point of view it is very easy to imagine that this may be helpful. It may seem to us that we are giving him more friends and more opportunities for pleasure; but the child himself is more likely to feel that he is being turned out of his home because he is jealous of the new brother or sister. He is in any case only too ready to feel that his own naughtinesses have made his mother prefer the new baby, and we may confirm this irremediably in his mind if we send him away at the time. It is true that we cannot always help doing so. If, for example, his mother is seriously ill, or there is no one at home to look after him, we may not be able to prevent this severe trial for the child. But it is another matter if we make such a mistake simply out of ignorance of what things may mean to the child himself, thus wasting our own goodwill and good efforts towards him.

Another major instance of an experience which every child has to go through, but which if possible should not be allowed to coincide with any further upheavals, is weaning. You will remember that Mrs. Klein emphasized this consideration in her chapter. Here again, if one is ignorant of the way the child's mind works, it may be easy to imagine it a suitable occasion to break the child off his attachment to the breast, when some other change has to be made, for instance, a holiday or a journey, a removal to another country, or a change of nurse. I would not say that such a situation would never be beneficial to any child, but the risk is only too great that the added disturbance and loss of, for example, a familiar nurse or familiar surroundings, will so intensify the child's feeling of loss and frustration in being taken from the breast that the whole foundations of his world will seem to him to be shaken. One instance in which this happened was very striking. A baby boy was fed at the breast until nine months, at which age the family had occasion to remove from England to another country. The mother took this opportunity of making the complete change from the breast to spoon and cup feeding, and this without any previous preparation. It is scarcely surprising to hear that the child was ill on the voyage, or that when the whole change of feeding was carried through in five weeks, three of which were occupied in a journey ending up in totally new surroundings, the child's desperate feeling of frustration and anxiety expressed itself in continual violent screaming which nothing could relieve for many months. Again, we may not always be able to avoid such coincidences. The illnesses of the child or grownups, external events over which we have no control, the birth of other children and other changes may create these difficulties for the child, even against our own good intentions. But if we do appreciate all that this may mean to him, we can help him so much more ; and may then take more trouble, as far as lies in our power, to arrange things better. It might, for example, be possible to time a change of nurse so that this did not coincide with an operation.

SUSAN ISAACS

Again, if we have to lose a nurse, we might arrange
the manner of her going so that the child should
not feel that it was his badness which had driven her
away.

It may, however, happen that circumstances are
too strong for us, and the child is thrown into an
acute emotional difficulty by some event—for example, the coincidence of his own teething or bad
temper with the illness of his mother or younger
baby. Whether from this or other causes it has to
be recognized that even when parents do their utmost and put the greatest amount of intelligence and
understanding into their care for their children,
some degree of emotional difficulty will arise from
time to time with every child. Emotional life is
so complicated, the problem of the conflict of love
and hate is so diverse and manifold, the child has to
struggle with such pressing desires and overwhelming fears at a time when his knowledge and control
are so weak. The interplay of inner and outer
forces is bound to bring about acute crises from
time to time, no matter how wise and loving we
are. Few if any children pass through the nursery
years without at least some temporary phase of
acute difficulty. I have already spoken of the help
which most mothers and nurses appear to gain
from the mere knowledge that these crises occur
even with normally developing children. In the
majority of cases the crisis will pass away, whether
it be acute phobias or feeding difficulties, tantrums
or dirtiness, provided that love and understanding
are given to the child. Fortunately, most children
have a great natural resilience, and there are always

224

inner tendencies within him making for harmony and health. But sometimes, even under the most favourable environments, his difficulties prove too acute or too persistent to yield to wise and humane education. The remaining function of the good parent is then to know when to call in outside help. Just as the wise mother knows when to send for the doctor and the nurse, because the knowledge and skill required to help the child through infectious illness or operation or digestive trouble is beyond her scope, so it is highly desirable that she should have sufficient wisdom and love to know when to call for the help of the psycho-analyst. And this may sometimes occur even with children of wise and healthy parents. We have seen that much more can be done than is generally realized at present to lessen the probability of such serious crises in development. Psycho-analytic work every day confirms the view that it is chiefly where the environment has been devoid of love and understanding that the most severe difficulties occur. In those cases where the child has become ill or unhappy *in spite of* sense and consideration on the part of the parent, it is very plain that he would have been very much worse if the parents had been inconsiderate or cruel. Nevertheless, it must be acknowledged that no one knows enough to produce health and happiness automatically. We have, therefore, to recognize that with *any* child there may come a situation in which the special technical help of analytic treatment is required, to safeguard against major breakdowns and failures in later life. There is no need for the parent to blame himself altogether when he is faced with the fact that his child is more unhappy or more difficult than he knows how to deal with. The interplay of psychic forces and external circumstances is extremely complex, and whilst we need every resource of our knowledge we can get, it is no use expecting miracles either from ourselves or from our children.

Psycho-analysts are the last people in the world to want to give the impression that they expect parents to be superhumanly loving and controlled and wise. Our study of children whose parents have attempted to be perfect has indeed convinced us how serious a mistake it may be to allow the responsibilities of parenthood to rest too heavily upon our shoulders. It is possible to overshoot the mark and undo the very good we aim at. Some parents feel such a sense of responsibility that they dare hardly look at or speak to their children. One mother of a little boy of fourteen months told me that so far she had not had a single day's happiness with her child, because she had been so overburdened by an awful sense of responsibility, and constantly thought how every word she said and every move she made might be fraught with infinite harm to him. And yet she appeared the very type of a loving and satisfied mother. She should have been this, but a little knowledge had, alas! made her too uneasy.

Those of us who come before the public to offer parents the fruits of our own experience do not do so in any light-hearted or dogmatic way. We know how many excellent parents there are who have never heard a word about psycho-analysis; and many who do not need to know anything about it, because their own natural relation with their children is balanced and harmonious. We know, too, that we may very readily disturb more than help those who come to us for knowledge and advice, if we overstress the responsibility of parenthood. We know so much of human nature that we would be the last people to suggest that parents should live only for their children and think of nothing but their children's welfare. The parent, the mother, the nurse, has her own emotional life to live, her own inner balance to maintain. If she shuts her eyes to this fact and blindly seeks to live only for her children, the natural equilibrium she herself needs will be gained at their expense in some other way. There is a limit beyond which none of us can go in self-sacrifice, a limit which is real for the child too. The parent who goes too far in the direction of self-sacrifice may injure rather than help the child. Every now and then in analytic work one sees the hatred and fear which parents who have sacrificed too much for the child may evoke in him. It is true that in the deepest layers of the child's mind he hates himself for having had to be the cause of so much self-sacrifice. But in his effective behaviour this will take the form of hatred and rejection of the parents, sometimes itself again covered up under cold and lifeless docility and devotion. Neither an ill-balanced subjection of the parents to the child nor the fantasy of being a perfect parent will in the end be as much aid to the child as a robust simplicity and a healthy balance between the parents' individuality and the child's.

At this point, then, we come back once more to

our initial question of how far it is possible for the nursery to be a community. It will be clear to you that I am suggesting that it is not only possible but highly desirable that the nursery should be a community. It should not be entirely " child-centred ", to use a phrase now in favour in educational circles. The school may and indeed in many respects should be " child-centred ", since it is created and maintained for the express purpose of educating children. The home, although in one sense so much more intimately at the service of the child, still cannot be completely centred in his needs. Father and mother, older brothers and sisters, have their claims there as much as the younger baby. Nor will it help the child to attempt to represent things to him otherwise.

Even in the nursery itself, as distinct from the larger setting of the home as a whole, this will hold true to some real extent. The nurse and the mother are persons, with personal rights and conveniences, and it is not desirable for the child that they should seem to sink every consideration to the child—or that they should feel that they ought to do so. If they seek to do this, the child will only be frightened. The expression of his love and his wishes to preserve and help those whom he loves will not be strengthened. Even for his sake, then, the nursery must be a community, a place where *every* member has privileges as well as responsibilities.

But of course the nursery is not and cannot be a community of equals. The function of the mother or nurse is to educate the child, to strengthen his constructive impulses by exercising her own knowledge and mature wisdom. Nurses and mothers are human, just as babies are, but their humanity is more developed and stable and, therefore, more free.

It is in those families where the parents are able to respect and serve both their own personalities and those of the children that we find a happy and ordered community life, one which increasingly equips the child for the varied functions of his life in the larger community outside the nursery and outside the home itself.

As another aspect of the nursery as a community of diverse individuals, I would finally suggest that whilst we may provide general conditions of life and training which are optimally favourable for the child's development, the actual solutions which he finds to his own psychic conflict cannot be determined by our preferences or our dictates. The child's gifts and interests, his tastes and loyalties, his type of character, the real personality which he will create for himself, even the degree or kind of neurosis which the child develops (and of course we all develop some), will always in the last resort be his own, not ours.

May I now remind you of the essential points made by the previous chapters as illustrating the various directions in which the nursery may become a true community?

Miss Sharpe emphasized the need for stability, not

only in the conscious plans, but also in the unconscious purposes of the parents, a stability which alone will make it possible for them to adapt to the special needs of the individual child at successive ages. She showed how rigid purposes, external to the child himself and imposed upon him by the parents' own conscious or unconscious needs, would fail to foster his development or to bring him ultimate happiness. Mrs. Klein mentioned the need to understand what the suckling situation in all its aspects of satisfaction and frustration, culminating in the final process of weaning, means to the child's feelings in his relation to his mother. She emphasized that the mother's own personality *as a whole* was as important to the child as the technique of weaning in the narrower sense. She showed how the mother who could herself find pleasure in the suckling and nursing of the child was all the more able to make him happy and contented, although her own pleasure should always be subordinated to the growth of the child and not be felt as an end in itself. The mother's happiness should lie in the child's life and development and in her own creative functioning towards that development.

Miss Searl, again, in referring to the many meanings which the child's questions may bear for him, asked the mother to let herself be alive to their emotional significance and the general background of feeling as well as to their factual content. She suggested that neither a mechanical reply of mere fact to the child's questions nor their emotional exploitation for our own purposes would ultimately help him, but only a kindly understanding of all the needs he expresses in his questions. In other words, we are able to answer the child's real questions only in so far as we are not afraid of his feelings and do not have to force them into the pattern of our own unconscious wishes and fears.

Once more, Dr. Middlemore asked us to allow the child his bodily pleasures and sensory experiences because of their essential aid to his development. She begged us not to be afraid of showing him un-equivocal and active affection, since the young child's delight in the bodily expressions of affection forms a solid basis for later good relations with other people, both sexual and social. In my own chapter on training in cleanliness I emphasized the desirability of avoiding rigid formulæ based upon theories of habit, and the unwisdom of forcing adult standards upon the young and immature child. I showed how help-ful it is to the child when the mother can await with love and confidence the normal ripening of his functions of control.

These detailed studies might all be summed up by saying that what seems to us psycho-analysts to be desirable is that the nursery should be a place where fathers and mothers, nurses and children alike, are real persons and allow each other to be real persons, with real pleasures and real activities ; where there is sincere emotional response, and feel-ings are not covered over or forced into rigid pat-terns by rules or formulæ. It is desirable that adults shall be themselves and allow children to be children. If they appreciate the real feelings and real personalities of their children they will not be afraid to demand that the children, too, shall recognize their personal reality and rights. Neither respect for abstract law or personal dignity, nor the unconscious sensual satisfaction of the parents, should be sought at the expense of the living growth of real children. Parents should keep their eyes on the child's future and have faith in his growth and development, whilst allowing him to live as fully and freely as he can on his own present level of love and achievement.

POSTSCRIPT

BY MELANIE KLEIN

RECENT research has added considerably to our knowledge of the earliest stage of infancy—roughly the first three or four months of life—and it is from this angle that I am writing this postscript.

As was described in detail in the chapter on Weaning, the very young infant's emotions are particularly powerful and are dominated by extremes. There are vigorous dividing processes between the two aspects (good and bad) of his first and most important object, the mother, and between his emotions (love and hatred) towards her. These divisions enable him to cope with his fears. The earliest fears derive from his aggressive impulses (which are easily stirred up by any frustration and discomfort) and take the form of feeling abandoned, injured, attacked—that is to say, intensely persecuted. Such persecutory fears, which focus on the mother, are prevalent in the infant until he develops a more integrated relation to her (and thereby to other people) which also implies an integration of his ego.

Recent investigations have been particularly concerned with the earliest stage of infancy. It has been recognised that the cleavage between love and hatred, usually described as a splitting of emotions, varies in intensity and takes many forms. These variations are bound up with the strength of persecutory fears in the infant. If splitting is excessive, the fundamentally important relation to the mother cannot be securely achieved and normal progress towards integration of the ego is disturbed. This may result in later mental illness. Another possible consequence is inhibition of intellectual development which may contribute to mental backwardness and—in extreme cases—to mental deficiency. Even in normal development there are temporary disturbances in the relation to the mother which are due to states of withdrawal both from her and from the experience of emotions. Should such states be too frequent or prolonged, they can be taken as an indication of abnormal development.

If the difficulties in the first phase are normally overcome, the infant is likely to succeed in dealing with the depressive feelings arising in the crucial stage which follows at the age of about four to six months.

The theoretical findings concerning the first year of life, which were derived from the analysis of young children (generally speaking from about two years onwards) have been confirmed in the analysis of older children and of adults as well. They have been increasingly applied to the observation of infantile behaviour, and the field has been widened to include even very young babies. Since this book first appeared, depressive feelings in young children have been more generally observed and recognised. Some of the phenomena now understood to be characteristic of the first three or four months of life are also in some degree observable. For instance, the states of withdrawal by which the infant cuts himself off from emotions imply an absence of response to his surroundings. In such states the infant may appear apathetic and without interest in his environment. This condition is more easily overlooked than other disturbances such as excessive crying, restlessness and refusal of food.

The growing understanding of the anxieties babies experience should also make it easier for all who have the care of young children to find ways in which these difficulties can be alleviated. Frustrations are up to a point unavoidable and the fundamental anxieties I have described cannot in any case be completely eradicated. A better understanding of the infant's emotional needs, however, is bound to influence favourably our attitude towards his problems and thereby help him on the road to stability. In expressing this hope I am summing up the main purpose of the present book.

LIST OF BOOKS

[This list makes no claim to completeness. As its title shows, it does not include papers published in the Quarterly Journals, as this would mean an enormous addition to its length, but the omission detracts from the value of the list. The books are selected as representatives of their class and for their suitability for the non-specialist reader. Most of them are not written by psycho-analysts and the views in them are not always those which a psycho-analyst would put forward, but they are included because they throw light on the mind of the child.

Notes are added in square brackets; the more popular expositions are marked with an asterisk.

J. R.]

S. BERNFELD. *The Psychology of the Infant.* London: Kegan Paul. 1929.

[A translation of " Psychologie des Säuglings ", first published in 1925. It is a clear exposition but naturally does not carry investigation so deeply as is done to-day.]

*K. BRIDGES. *Social and Emotional Development of the Pre-School Child.* London: Kegan Paul. 1931.

[A study of the behaviour of a group of children in the nursery school, which attempts to arrive at a scale for measuring how far the social development of particular children is normal for their age.]

*CHARLOTTE BÜHLER. *The First Year of Life.* London: John Day. 1930.

[The feature of this book is the hour by hour, minute by minute observation of the babies who were being watched. The facts given in this book will come as a surprise to many who think that they have been fairly good observers of children !]

*L. Chaloner. *Modern Babies and Nurseries.* Oxford University Press. 1929.

[A simple and useful study of the child in the nursery.]

*W. de Kok. *New Babes for Old.* London: Gollancz. 1932. Pp. 186.

[A simple account of the author's own two children, with many practical hints as to the best way of dealing with emotional problems.]

S. Freud. *Introductory Lectures on Psycho-Analysis.* Translated by Joan Riviere. London: Allen & Unwin. Revised Ed. 1929.

[A classical series of lectures. The best single introduction to the subject of psycho-analysis.]

S. Freud. *The Ego and the Id.* London: Hogarth Press. 1927.

[A landmark in the study of the unconscious basis of the moral elements in human personality.]

A. Gesell. *Infancy and Human Growth.* London: Macmillan. 1928.

[A technical account of researches into the course of mental development during the first five years, with an attempt to arrive at definite norms of mental growth for successive ages. Very important in its own field.]

F. L. Goodenough. *Anger in Young Children.* University of Minnesota Press. 1931.

[A study of the frequency of tantrums in young children at different ages, the situations which give rise to such tantrums, and the best methods of dealing with them.]

*V. Hazlitt. *Psychology of Infancy.* London: Methuen. 1933.

[A clear account of mental development during the first three years, showing the growth of the child's perceptions and understanding of the world.]

O. C. Irwin. *The Activities of Infants during the First Ten Days.* Clark University Press. Genetic Psychology Monographs, Vol. VIII. 1930.

[An experimental study of the learning capacity of infants. Shows that even in the first ten days there are considerable differences between one child and another.]

*SUSAN ISAACS. *The Psychological Aspects of Child Development.* London: University of London Institute of Education and Evans Bros. 1935. Pp. 45.

> [A very condensed but clear account of current knowledge and technique; it is comparable to a key map, which is of use in fitting together more detailed surveys into a comprehensible whole.]

*SUSAN ISAACS. *The Nursery Years.* London: Routledge. 1932. Revised Ed.

> [A very simple and practical account of the child's mental development and his emotional and intellectual needs during the first five years. It offers practical suggestions on education, play material, etc.]

SUSAN ISAACS. *Intellectual Growth in Young Children. Social Development in Young Children.* London: Routledge. 1933.

> [These two volumes are based upon detailed records of the behaviour of a group of intelligent young children in a nursery school. The first volume describes the experiments, questions, discussions and arguments, and practical interests of the children, and the growth of their understanding of the physical world from these experiences. The second one describes their friendships and quarrels, and development in social co-operation and their relations to adults; and then offers a psychoanalytic interpretation of these different sorts of behaviour. It ends with the application of these psychological findings to the problems of education.]

*ERNEST JONES. *Psycho-Analysis.* London: Benn. Benn's Sixpenny Series.] 1928. Pp. 80.

> [A simple and clear account of the theory and method of psycho-analysis, showing its applications to medicine, education, etc.]

MELANIE KLEIN. *The Psycho-Analysis of Children.* London: Hogarth Press. 1932. Pp. 393.

> [This is the classical book on the psycho-analytical researches into the mind of the child. It has done more than any other in the last ten years to revolutionize our concept of unconscious mental processes.]

MARGARET LOWENFELD. *Play in Childhood.* London:
Gollancz. 1935. Pp. 345.

> [Valuable for its description of the way in which ordinary
> domestic and toy-shop objects can be used by the child to
> express his fantasies; the elaboration of the theories derived
> from the observation of the play is concerned almost exclusively
> with the conscious levels of the mind.]

G. MURPHY and L. C. MURPHY. *Experimental Social Psychology.* New York and London. 1931. Harper Bros.

> [A very comprehensive survey of all the facts of social behaviour
> in children of different ages, as these facts are gathered by
> objective, descriptive and experimental methods; full of the
> most useful and interesting facts, although it does not go below
> the surface.]

*J. PIAGET. *The Child's Conception of the World.* London:
Kegan Paul. 1930.

> [A study of the child's beliefs about such things as dreams,
> names, the nature of life, and the origins of natural phenomena
> such as lakes, rivers, the sun and the moon. Full of interesting
> material, showing how differently the world presents itself to the
> child and the adult.]

K. C.-PRATT, H. K. NELSON, and K. H. SUN. *The Behaviour
of the New-Born Infant.* Ohio: State University Studies
Contributions to Psychology. 1930.

> [An exact experimental study of the behaviour of the new-born
> infant in response to changes of light, temperature, contact, etc.]

M. M. SHIRLEY. *The First Two Years.* Vols. I, II, and III.
University of Minnesota Press. 1933.

> [A detailed scientific study, from the point of view of the
> psychologist, a doctor and an anatomist, of the development
> of twenty-five babies. Vol. I deals with postural control and
> learning to walk; Vol. II, with manipulative skills and
> language; Vol. III, with social responses and individual
> differences in personality.]

KARIN STEPHEN. *Psycho-Analysis and Medicine.* Cambridge
University Press. 1933.

> [An introduction to psycho-analytic theory through a series of
> case studies; intended mainly for medical students.]

LIST OF BOOKS

*L. WAGONER. *Development of Learning in Young Children.*
London : McGraw-Hill. 1933. Pp. xiv + 322.

[A very clear and useful account of the spontaneous learning
of the young child, his interests, the development of bodily
skills, language and social behaviour.]

R. W. WASHBURN. *The Smiling and Laughing of Infants in the
First Year of Life.* Clark University Press. Genetic
Psychology Monographs. Vol. VI. 1929.

[A study of the frequency of smiling and laughing at different
ages during the first year and the situations in which these
occur.]

D. W. WINNICOTT. *Clinical Notes on Disorders of Childhood.*
London : Heinemann. 1931.

[A valuable study, based on the clinical experience of the
doctor, of the psychological factors in the common ailments of
early childhood.]

ADDITIONS (JANUARY 1952)

JOHN BOWLBY. *Forty-four Juvenile Thieves: Their Characters
and Home Life.* London: Bailliere, Tindall & Cox. 1946.

[A survey which demonstrates the correlation between early
separation from the mother or her substitute and the delinquent
affectionless character.]

*JOHN BOWLBY. *Maternal Care and Mental Health.* Geneva :
World Health Organisation. 1951.

[Report prepared on behalf of the W.H.O. as a contribution to
the United Nations programme for the welfare of homeless
children.]

DOROTHY BURLINGHAM and ANNA FREUD. *Young Children in
Wartime.* London : Allen & Unwin. 1942.

[A description of the Hampstead Nurseries and the reactions of
the children to their wartime experiences, in the light of the
authors' theories about the emotional development of the
child.]

*DOROTHY BURLINGHAM and ANNA FREUD. *Infants Without Families.* London : Allen & Unwin. 1944.

> [An account of the behaviour of children in a wartime residential nursery, showing the value to the child's growth in personality of small family units within the institution.]

*AUDREY DAVIDSON and JUDITH FAY. *Phantasy in Childhood.* In preparation. Routledge & Kegan Paul.

> [An attempt to express some of Melanie Klein's theories in non-technical language, and to show both how they are repeatedly borne out in the day-to-day behaviour of children, and how helpful some knowledge of the phantasies described by her can be from a practical point of view.]

RUTH GRIFFITHS. *Imagination in Early Childhood.* London : Kegan Paul. 1945.

> [An investigation into the imaginative life of children in infant schools in England and Australia, by means of drawings and conversations arising out of them.]

*SUSAN ISAACS, JOAN RIVIERE and ELLA FREEMAN SHARPE. *Fatherless Children.* London : New Education Fellowship Monograph No. 2. Pushkin Press. 1945.

> [A short account of the significance and importance of the father, and of the particular difficulties experienced by the child and his mother in the event of his death.]

SUSAN ISAACS. *Childhood and After.* London : Routledge & Kegan Paul. 1948.

> [A collection of papers varying from technical psycho-analytic studies to simple essays addressed to a lay public, the common thread running through them being the feelings, phantasies and needs of the child, which must be appreciated in order to understand the adult.]

*SUSAN ISAACS. *Troubles of Children and Parents.* London : Methuen. 1948.

> [A selection of letters written by mothers and nurses to *The Nursery World* seeking advice over problems with their children and the replies they received from Mrs Isaacs under her pseudonym of Ursula Wise.]

*MELANIE KLEIN and JOAN RIVIERE. *Love, Hate and Reparation.* London : Psycho-Analytical Epitomes No. 2. Hogarth Press. 1937.

> [A very clear and simple account of the child's conflicts over his love and hatred, exemplified in the everyday behaviour of adults.]

242

LIST OF BOOKS

MELANIE KLEIN. *Contributions to Psycho-Analysis, 1921–45.* London : Hogarth Press. 1948.

[An account of the development of the author's work over a period of twenty-five years. The papers are complementary to the *Psycho-Analysis of Children* and show how the author reached her conclusions and on what lines her work was continued.]

MELANIE KLEIN, PAULA HEIMANN, SUSAN ISAACS, and JOAN RIVIERE. *Developments in Psycho-Analysis.* In preparation. Hogarth Press.

[A survey of the most recent progress in theory clarifying some of the conclusions propounded in the *Psycho-Analysis of Children* and in *Contributions to Psycho-Analysis.* This volume also contains instances of the observation of very young children.]

*MERELL P. MIDDLEMORE. *The Nursing Couple.* London : Hamish Hamilton Medical Books. 1941.

[A study of the reactions of newborn infants and their mothers to the suckling situation.]

MARGARET RIBBLE. *The Rights of Infants.* New York : Columbia University Press. 1943.

[A study showing the importance of mothering to the baby, and the close interrelation between emotional and physical development, with special emphasis on the value of the stimulation of personal contact from the physiological point of view.]

ELLA FREEMAN SHARPE. *Collected Papers on Psycho-Analysis.* London : Hogarth Press. 1950.

[A collection of papers on the technique and theory of psychoanalysis, and on literary interpretation.]

*D. W. WINNICOTT. *Getting to Know Your Baby.* London : Pamphlet William Heinemann Medical Books. 1945.

[A discussion in simple language of infant feelings, and the importance of the earliest relationship between mother and baby.]

*D. W. WINNICOTT. *The Ordinary Devoted Mother.* London: Pamphlet distributed privately. 87 Chester Square, S.W.1. 1949.

[Broadcast talks to mothers about the psychological importance of a baby's experiences, and the help a good mother can give him.]

243